MW01002437

the
WHEAT
FREE

Diet

&

Cookbook

DELICIOUS
WHEAT FREE
RECIPES

Rockridge Press

CONTENTS

Introduction 1

Chapter 1: Wheat: The Good, the Bad, and the Ugly 3

What Is Wheat? 4

The History of Wheat 5

Should We Call It Frankenwheat? 6

Chapter 2: The Dangers of Wheat 9

Wheat, Obesity, Insulin, and Diabetes 10

Wheat and the Immune System 12

Wheat and Mental/Emotional Health 13

Wheat as an Addictive Drug 14

Chapter 3: The Benefits of a Wheat-Free Lifestyle 15

Aging 16

Brain Function 18

Insulin 20

pH Balance 21

Skin Health 22

Weight 24

Wheat Allergies 25

Gluten Intolerance 26

Celiac Disease 27

Chapter 4: Living Wheat-Free   **30**

   Wheat-Free, Gluten-Free, Grain-Free:
   What's the Difference?   30

   Embracing the Wheat-Free Lifestyle   31

   What to Eat   32

   What to Avoid   38

   Alternative Ingredients   41

Chapter 5: Transitioning into the Wheat-Free Diet   **42**

   10 Tips for a Successful Transition   42

   Wheat Withdrawal and How to Survive It   46

   Wheat-Free Diet Seven-Day Meal Plan   47

Chapter 6: Wheat-Free Diet   **55**

  Snacks and Appetizers   **55**

   Smoked Salmon-Stuffed Tomatoes   55

   Black Bean Hummus Dip   56

   Mediterranean Salad   57

   Mushroom-Stuffed Mushrooms   58

   Spicy Crab and Cucumber Canapés   59

   Seafood-Stuffed Shells   60

   Spinach and Orange Salad with
   Sesame-Lime Dressing   61

   Crispy Kale Chips   62

   Pear and Prosciutto Packets   63

   Spicy Roasted Nuts   64

  Breakfast   **65**

   Mushroom and Pesto Omelet   65

   Hearty Hot Flax Cereal   66

Morning Latte Smoothie 67

Quinoa Breakfast Parfait 68

Sweet and Spicy Pumpkin Bread 69

Savory Morning Hash 71

Fresh Breakfast Scramble 72

Southwestern Breakfast Skillet 73

Apple-Cinnamon Protein Shake 74

Special Steak and Eggs 75

Lunch **76**

Simply Good Chicken Noodle Soup 76

Philly Lettuce Wraps 77

Asian Noodle Bowl 78

Mediterranean Grilled Chicken Salad 79

Egg Salad in Avocadoes 80

Creamy Tomato Soup 81

Easy Spinach Quiche 82

Roasted Vegetable Soup 83

Shrimp and Avocado Platter 85

Noodles with Ham and Peas 86

Dinner **87**

Pecan-Crusted Flounder 87

Pork Loin with Roasted Sweet Potato Strips 89

Orange and Ginger Flank Steak Stir-Fry 91

Garlic and Herb Roasted Chicken 93

Shirataki Shrimp Scampi 95

Wine-Braised Cabbage Rolls 96

Hearty Beef and Vegetable Soup 98

Shrimp and Asparagus Pasta   99

Spicy Beef and Peppers   100

Dilly-Orange Sole Steamed in Foil   101

Dessert   **102**

No-Flour Rich Chocolate Cake   102

Pecan-Apple Tart   104

Creamy Coconut Rice Pudding   105

Warm Peach Parfaits   106

Individual Pumpkin-Pecan Custards   107

Creamy Espresso Mousse   108

Strawberry-Pineapple Sorbet   109

Peanut Butter-Raisin Cookies   110

Very Berry Dessert   111

Frothy Chocolate Milkshakes   112

Conclusion   **113**

References   **114**

INTRODUCTION

For years, we've been told that including grains in our diet was essential for good health. In the last two decades or so, Americans have been admonished to include as many grains in their diets as possible, especially whole grains. Since wheat is the most common grain in the American diet, it follows that most of those whole-grain foods would contain wheat.

This should be a good thing; but perhaps it isn't.

Research from more than one scientific circle indicates that our consumption of wheat is directly responsible for several conditions and diseases in the United States, including type 2 diabetes, obesity, high blood pressure, insulin resistance, arterial disease, and many others. This is in addition to the problems associated with celiac disease, a condition that damages the lining of the small intestine due to a sensitivity to gluten, which is a protein composite found in wheat and other related grains.

In the 1970s, Dr. Robert Atkins released *Dr. Atkins' Diet Revolution*, the first of several books warning of the effects of a high-carbohydrate diet. His and other low-carb diets advised that flour-based foods such as bread and pasta were too large a part of the American diet and could be blamed for much of the obesity Americans were facing. While the original Atkins diet has been revised several times, the low-carb movement has gained respect and credibility.

Just a few years ago, the Paleo diet generated a great deal of attention with the premise that humans were not actually designed to consume grains; that our digestive systems had not adapted to eating them and our consumption of them was making us overweight and ill.

More recently, William Davis, MD, a cardiologist, released his book, *Wheat Belly: Lose the Wheat, Lose the Weight, and Find Your Path Back to Health*, in which he shared his own research. What Dr. Davis revealed was that while humans have adapted somewhat to eating grains, we were able to digest only the grains (in particular, the wheat) that were grown up until the mid-twentieth century. Since that time, he asserts, the wheat grown in the United States has been genetically modified so much that our bodies haven't had time to adapt to it. Not only that, but he explains that those modifications have resulted in a wheat product that is unsafe for us to eat. *(Davis 2011)*

The scientists behind the Paleo diet, Dr. Davis, and many other researchers agree that removing wheat from our diets can prevent or reverse many of the health problems that have become nearly epidemic in America.

Going on a wheat-free diet may seem impossible; however, doing so can mean living a longer, healthier, leaner life. Plus, "wheat-free" doesn't mean "taste-free"! You don't have to give up your favorite foods, such as pastas, breads, cereals, cookies, cakes, and many others. There are great recipes, such as the ones in this book, that replace the wheat without giving up on the taste and the texture. And once you've been on the wheat-free diet for a few weeks, the results, along with the wonderful foods that you are eating, will more than make up for the loss of wheat.

1

WHEAT: THE GOOD, THE BAD, AND THE UGLY

I t's not enough to say that wheat is bad for you and you shouldn't eat it, especially when wheat-based products make up such a large part of the American diet. It's important to know exactly what wheat is, how it came to be so important in the human diet, and how eating it affects our bodies and our health.

Making good nutritional decisions and healthful changes requires knowledge. Too often, fad diets advise people to cut out whole groups of foods in an effort to lose weight, while brushing over the fact that those foods provide important nutrients.

The wheat-free diet isn't just about losing weight; it's also about improving your current health and preventing future problems, such as heart disease and diabetes. Therefore, it's important to understand the science behind the wheat-free diet, rather than simply rushing into a wheat-free lifestyle in the hopes of dropping the pounds. Most people will lose weight on the diet as a result of cutting many unhealthful foods from their menus, but this weight loss should be seen as a wonderful bonus of the diet, not the main focus.

What Is Wheat?

The crop that we know as wheat is a cereal grain that originally grew wild as a plant similar to grasses. The part that we eat is at the top of the plant and is known as the grain. The whole grain is milled to separate the endosperm, bran, and germ. The stem or stalk (what we know as straw) is inedible.

The endosperm alone is ground to make white flour, while the bran and germ are reserved for other uses. In whole-grain flour, the wheat has been ground with the bran and germ intact.

There are several different species of wheat cultivated today. Some of the more common types are semolina, durum, and soft and hard winter wheat. They differ in the amount of protein and gluten they contain, and some are preferred over others for specific uses.

Not Bread Alone

When most people think of wheat, they think of bread. Breads are one of the most common products made with wheat; however, a vast number of foods contain wheat flour. Most pasta is made from wheat, as are many cereals. Even cereals that don't contain wheat as a main ingredient still use wheat as filler.

Wheat is also used in products that, on the surface, seem to have nothing to do with flour or grain. Flavored coffees, for instance, usually contain a derivative of wheat. So do some herbal teas. Many types of vodka are distilled from wheat. A huge number of artificial colorings and flavorings are derived from wheat.

DID YOU KNOW? *Many people committed to lowering their sugar intake are still eating "healthful" wheat products such as whole-wheat bread even though one teaspoon of table sugar has a glycemic index of 59, while a slice of whole-wheat bread has a glycemic index of 72!*

As you can see, the bread basket is not the only place that you will find wheat, and there's far more of it in your diet than you might think. Even if you don't each much bread, cake, or cereal, your wheat intake is probably quite significant.

If You Are What You Eat, You'd Better Understand Your Food

There are two key arguments against eating wheat. One is that our bodies weren't actually designed to eat wheat and haven't yet fully adapted to it. The other is that the wheat we're eating has changed so drastically over the last fifty years that it's dangerous, whether we adapt to eating it or not.

This is why it's so important to know how our bodies process and use wheat and to understand how the wheat we eat today differs from the wheat our ancestors consumed. To do that, we need to understand the history of wheat as a food, from ten thousand years ago right up to the twenty-first century.

The History of Wheat

The first documented evidence of human beings using wheat for food involves the Natufians, a semi-nomadic people that lived in the areas now known as Syria, Lebanon, Israel, Iraq, and Jordan. Archeologists have found among the ruins of Natufian homes remains of harvested einkorn wheat (the original wild variety of the grain) as well as harvesting tools.

Wheat is easily self-pollinated, and einkorn wheat eventually bred with other grasses and formed a new variety of wheat called *emmer*. This variety was one of the most common cultivated for food for several centuries, but it eventually changed as well, through a combination of intentional breeding and self-pollination. What resulted was a variety of wheat known as *Triticum aestivum*.

Triticum aestivum became the most commonly cultivated wheat and the one on which whole civilizations depended. Cities were built around agriculture that consisted largely of wheat, and grain was as good as cash in many societies. Grain became a true staple, with the poorest people often depending on bread for their survival.

Triticum aestivum evolved very little between several thousand years ago and the latter half of the twentieth century. In the mid to late 1900s, as agriculture (and wheat crops) became big business, agricultural scientists and researchers began looking for ways to increase wheat yields without increasing acreage. And they were quite successful. In fact, wheat yields on the average farm acre are now *ten times* what they were just one hundred years ago. So how do you make a grain yield ten times greater?

This was accomplished through a combination of new chemical fertilizers, the developments of new pesticides, and the breeding of new types of wheat by modifying the wheat's genetics. This last method is one that impacts our health the most today.

Should We Call It Frankenwheat?

To understand how wheat has been changed and how that change affects us, a simple understanding about wheat genetics is needed. Wheat has one of the most complex genetic makeups in the natural world. In human beings, the forty-six chromosomes of each parent are blended to create forty-six chromosomes in their child. But in wheat (like some other plants), the chromosomes of each "parent" are added to make a new plant. In other words, the genetic makeup of wheat is cumulative. This ability to add chromosomes is called *polyploidy*, and it doesn't occur in animals or people. *(Shewry 2009)*

Einkorn wheat started out with only fourteen chromosomes. When it mated with wild goat grass, the resulting strain was emmer wheat, which had twenty-eight chromosomes. Sometime prior to even the

Old Testament era, emmer mated with another grass to form *Triticum aestivum*, which had forty-two chromosomes. *(Shewry 2009)*

As we said earlier, *Triticum aestivum* changed very little over the ensuing years. It remained largely the same until genetic modification and hybridization became far better understood and more widely practiced. The fact that wheat has such a complex genetic code actually makes it quite flexible, genetically speaking.

Those agricultural scientists interested in increasing wheat yields quickly turned to altering the actual genetic code of wheat to make it more resistant to disease, more tolerant of heat and drought, and a more compact plant.

The problem is that all of this genetic engineering produced a type of wheat whose proteins, gluten content, and enzymes are very different from *Triticum aestivum*. In fact, each type of new wheat is also different from its parents. In testing one particular strain, researchers found that 95 percent of the resulting genes matched those of its parent plants, but 5 percent of the genes found were completely new. *(Song et al. 2009)*

To understand where this is heading, imagine that through genetic engineering, new human genes were created. What if people suddenly had a new organ or a new limb? How many new parts would humans need to have before they became another species altogether? It may sound silly, and it is an exaggerated example, but the principle is very close to the truth, and the wheat we consume today is a sort of "Frankenwheat" that bears little resemblance to the wheat our ancestors ate.

Scarier than Frankenwheat?

What makes all this genetic tampering all the more alarming is that while it was taking place, no one was interested in finding out whether these new strains of wheat were actually safe for human consumption. Because these new genetic structures resulted in something that could still be classified as wheat and because being able to grow more food in less space was considered such a good thing, no one was much interested in whether it was actually healthful.

One of the questions that has been raised in recent years is why there have been so many more health problems associated with wheat in the last few decades. Has the incidence of celiac disease skyrocketed or was it just misdiagnosed in the past? Why didn't the wheat-eating population of the 1940s have as many problems with obesity as we now do? Why are breads and pastas and cereals being blamed for blood-sugar problems as much as sugar is?

In the next section, I'll explain in greater detail how the "new" wheat dramatically impacts our health in so many ways—from psychological and mental issues to arterial disease and diabetes.

2

THE DANGERS OF WHEAT

What makes the eating of wheat and the nature of the wheat we're eating so important is that it impacts so many of our body's systems.

The dangers of eating today's wheat don't stop at weight gain or even celiac disease. Its properties have an adverse effect on our digestive systems, our heart health, our immune systems, and even our mental and emotional health. What's more, there's now solid evidence that certain properties of wheat actually promote an addiction to the stuff.

Smoking has been shown unequivocally to cause lung cancer, stroke, emphysema, and heart disease. It has also been proven to be extremely addictive, making smokers crave the very thing that has been shown to be a danger to their health.

Perhaps twenty years from now, wheat will be considered on the same par as cigarettes.

In this chapter, we'll take a closer look at the specific ways that eating wheat, especially the wheat being produced today, affects the various systems of the body and why it's so important to cut wheat from the diet.

Wheat, Obesity, Insulin, and Diabetes

Obesity, the insulin response and our sensitivity to it, and type 2 diabetes are usually considered three separate health issues, so it would make sense to discuss them separately, as well. However, they're so closely intertwined that it's almost impossible to do so.

Wheat and Obesity

One of the more obvious impacts of wheat on weight and obesity are the calories involved with eating wheat products.

Think about the wheat products that you commonly consume. You're not just eating bread, but pasta, breakfast cereals, pizza, cakes, cookies, muffins, and so much more. All of these foods typically contain a huge number of calories, but very little nutrition.

For example, a large cinnamon raisin bagel has about 365 calories. A wheat hamburger bun has about 180. That big blueberry muffin from the coffee shop weighs in at around 380 calories. The microwavable macaroni and cheese you love packs 340 calories (per serving, *not* per package). Three of those homemade chocolate-chip cookies your coworker brought to the office will add about 230 calories to your daily intake.

As you can see (and probably already suspected), wheat foods add a lot of calories to your daily diet; but the calories in and of themselves are not the whole problem.

The carbohydrates in wheat are digested very quickly and turned into glucose. When there is glucose present in your bloodstream, your body responds by secreting insulin. Insulin's job is to get that glucose out of your bloodstream and into your cells, where it can be used as energy. The more glucose in your blood, the more insulin is secreted. However, if your body doesn't require all of the glucose present, it stores the excess as visceral fat, which is a layer of fat surrounding your organs. This is different from subcutaneous fat, which is the fat just below your skin.

There are several significant dangers of excess visceral fat. Aside from the added strain that it puts on your heart, visceral fat disrupts normal hormone balance and function so much that it has been labeled as an actual endocrine gland.

Research suggests that fat cells—particularly abdominal fat cells—are biologically active. It's appropriate to think of fat as an endocrine organ or gland, producing hormones and other substances that can profoundly affect our health. . . . Although scientists are still deciphering the roles of individual hormones, it's becoming clear that excess body fat, especially abdominal fat, disrupts the normal balance and functioning of these hormones. **(Harvard School of Public Health 2007)**

How does this affect your body? Several hormones are known to be disrupted, including leptin, ghrelin, insulin, and cortisol. Leptin and ghrelin tell you when you're hungry and when you're full. Insulin, of course, moves glucose into the cells or stores it as fat. Cortisol is a stress hormone that stimulates the storage of fat around the abdomen.

The effects on insulin, however, are extremely troubling to the medical community because they have far-reaching consequences.

Wheat, Insulin, and Insulin Resistance

Continued exposure to excess insulin in the bloodstream results in continued storage of visceral fat. These two problems often lead to a decreased sensitivity to insulin itself. The cells don't respond to insulin the way they're supposed to and less glucose is moved from the blood to the cells. This is what's called *insulin resistance,* and the excess blood glucose is known as *high blood sugar.*

When insulin resistance goes uncorrected, it very often leads to type 2 diabetes.

Wheat, Type 2 Diabetes, and Heart Disease

According to Centers for Disease Control and Prevention, in 1980 only about four hundred thousand new cases of type 2 diabetes were diagnosed each year. Every year since 2008, 1.8 million new cases have been diagnosed annually.

The startling increase in new type 2 diabetes cases lends weight to Dr. William Davis's assertion that the increase in obesity and type 2 diabetes can be tied to the genetic modification of wheat that began in the 1980s.

Type 2 diabetes can be prevented and can be reversed, but left untreated, it leads to very serious health issues.

According to the American Heart Association, people with type 2 diabetes are two- to four-times more likely to have a stroke and two- to four-times more likely to die of heart disease. Type 2 diabetes can also lead to kidney damage or kidney failure, diseases of the eye and loss of vision, and nerve damage.

As you can see, wheat and its effects on obesity, insulin, and type 2 diabetes are closely related and actually create a very dangerous cycle. When you couple this with the fact that certain properties in wheat have actually been shown to be addictive (more on that later in this chapter), this cycle becomes even harder to avoid or break.

Wheat and the Immune System

Researchers are just beginning to understand the effects of wheat and gluten on the body's immune system. While we've known for some time now that gluten triggers serious inflammation in the body of a person with celiac disease, we are just now learning that the immune systems of people *without* celiac are also affected.

In people suffering from celiac disease, certain parts of the immune system are triggered by antibodies to gluten and the inflammation that results. In gluten-sensitive people, there are antibodies present, but not to the same extent. In a recent study published in the *Journal of the American Medical Association*, researchers reported that people who had not been diagnosed with either celiac or gluten sensitivity still had a generalized immune response to gluten. This response is called *innate immunity*, and it can cause many of the same symptoms as celiac. The resulting inflammation can also cause the same problems, such as heart disease. (*Ludvigsson et al. 2009*)

Wheat and Mental/Emotional Health

You probably don't think of mental or emotional health issues as being connected to the consumption of wheat, but that connection was first established back in the 1960s by a psychiatrist named Dr. F. Curtis Dohan. During World War II, Dr. Dohan had noticed that when wheat rations were cut and bread and wheat products were unavailable, far fewer servicemen were diagnosed with schizophrenia.

Later on, while Dr. Dohan was working in a mental hospital, he conducted a study of schizophrenics in his care. When wheat was removed from their diets, these patients exhibited far fewer symptoms in just four weeks. When the patients were allowed to have wheat once again, the symptoms returned. (*Costa and Trabucchi 1980*)

Since then, studies have been done on various mental and emotional conditions and their relationships to eating wheat.

In a study of fifty-five Dutch autistic children, a gluten-free diet was shown to lessen several symptoms, despite the fact that the children were not known to suffer from celiac disease. (*Whiteley et al. 2010*)

Similar results have been reported in studies of both adults and children with attention-deficit/hyperactivity disorder (ADHD).

Wheat as an Addictive Drug

We've heard for several years that carbohydrates can be addicting, and many people have diagnosed themselves as being "carb addicts." This has often been blamed on the energy/fatigue cycle caused by eating sugary carbs. You eat a high-carb, high-sugar snack to get a lift, experience a quick burst of energy, and then a quick crash before having another high-carb, high-sugar snack to combat it.

But research now shows that wheat actually acts as an addictive drug and this may be where real carb addiction actually comes from.

When your body digests wheat, the proteins in the wheat are converted into *polypeptides*, which are shorter proteins. These polypeptides are called *exorphins* and they produce a high similar to the one you get from the endorphins produced by exercise or sex. This high comes from the binding of the exorphins to the *opioid* (morphine) receptors of the brain. The exorphins that come from wheat proteins are called *gluteomorphins* because they come from gluten and behave very similar to morphine, including causing addiction to them. *(Zioudrou, Streaty, and Klee 1979)*

If you recall from Chapter 1, the wheat being grown today has much more protein in it because of the genetic modifications that have been done. More protein equals more gluteomorphins. More gluteomorphins equal more addiction.

DID YOU KNOW? *In the study on wheat and diabetes that was published in the* Journal of the American Medical Association, *it was reported that hidden gluten sensitivity (elevated antibodies are present but the patient has not been diagnosed with celiac disease) was shown to increase a person's risk of death by 35 to 75 percent, mostly by causing heart disease and cancer.* (Ludvigsson et al. 2009)

When you consider that wheat and gluten have been linked to obesity, type 2 diabetes, heart disease, and even mental and emotional disorders, it's very disturbing to know that wheat can be addicting. Fortunately, that addiction can be broken by adopting a wheat-free lifestyle.

3

THE BENEFITS OF A WHEAT-FREE LIFESTYLE

To some extent, we are a benefits-driven society. Sometimes, the possible benefits of a lifestyle change are more motivating than the possible bad effects of not making that change.

While some people are motivated to exercise because being sedentary can lead to weight gain, bone loss, and heart disease; others are motivated to exercise because it makes them feel good, helps them to enjoy more of the foods they love, and makes their clothes fit better.

While some people are motivated to quit smoking because cigarettes cause cancer and stroke; others are more motivated by the fact that quitting will save them money, make their family happy, and help them to enjoy their favorite physical activities again.

Making the change to a wheat-free diet doesn't just help us to avoid the diseases and disorders associated with eating wheat; it also brings many other benefits, such as weight loss, increased bone strength, clearer skin, and better focus and memory.

In this chapter, we'll take a side-by-side look at some negative impacts of eating wheat and the positive impacts of living wheat-free.

Aging

For some time, people with type 2 diabetes have been used in studies on advanced aging. When most people think of the signs of aging, they think of wrinkles, age spots, and other visible evidence. What we're talking about here, though, is the presence of conditions in young people that are normally associated with the elderly.

Type 2 diabetics have been studied so often because of the presence in their bodies of a high number of AGEs, or advanced glycation end-products. Glycation and its effect on the body are explained very well by Dr. Ayla Wilson in an article on wheat and advanced aging.

A high carbohydrate diet causing elevated blood glucose levels leads to a process called glycation. Glycation occurs when a sugar group attaches onto a protein within the body, leading to the formation of an Advanced Glycation Endproduct or AGE. This can occur in the arteries, eyes, kidneys, skin, liver, nerves, and virtually anywhere in the body. Everyone has some AGEs, but high levels are a sign of accelerated aging. AGEs lead to degenerative conditions such as cataracts, dementia, kidney disease, clogged arteries, saggy/wrinkled skin, and arthritis. Once formed, AGEs are irreversible, but changes can be made to slow AGE production. (Wilson 2011)

The buildup of AGEs is not restricted to diabetics. Continued high blood sugar caused by eating high-carb foods is enough to cause the formation of AGEs in people without diabetes.

Where does wheat specifically come in? Dr. William Davis explains:

The "complex" carbohydrate contained in wheat is the unique variety of amylopectin, amylopectin A, a form distinct from amylopectin in other carbohydrates such as black beans and bananas. The amylopectin of wheat is the form most readily digested by the enzyme amylase, thus explaining the greater blood sugar–increasing property of wheat products. The more rapid and efficient digestion of wheat amylopectin means higher blood sugars over the ensuing two hours after consumption of wheat products, which in turn means greater triggering of AGE formation. If AGE formation was a contest, wheat would win nearly all the time, beating out other carbohydrate sources such as apples, oranges, sweet potatoes, ice cream, and chocolate bars. (Davis 2011)

Symptoms of Advanced Aging

It's clear that eating wheat contributes enormously to the formation and high accumulation of AGEs in the body. Most of the physical symptoms are related to diseases and conditions such as type 2 diabetes, kidney disease or kidney failure, cataracts or blindness, and other serious ailments. However, the compromised function of the body's major organs can also result in dry, uneven skin, premature wrinkling, joint pain, and even early symptoms of Alzheimer's disease or dementia.

DID YOU KNOW? *AGEs can be measured by a simple blood test called the Hemoglobin A1c. It measures AGE production over a period of 60-90 days, and you can take the test every three months to track AGE activity. A lower HbA1c means that blood sugar is under control, AGE production is minimized, and accelerated aging is not occurring.* (Wilson 2011)

The Wheat-Free Diet's Impact on Advanced Aging

Many of the advanced aging issues are directly related to the development of type 2 diabetes. Many respected studies have shown that diet modification, weight loss, and exercise can not only prevent type 2 diabetes in those diagnosed with metabolic syndrome (prediabetes) but can also reverse diabetes in those who already have the disease.

While most researchers agree that AGEs cannot be eliminated from the body once there, going on a wheat-free diet now can slow the accumulation of AGEs and prevent many of the problems associated with them.

Brain Function

There are several alarming neurological effects of eating wheat, aside from the fogginess, lack of concentration, and poor memory associated with the blood sugar crash that follows a high-carb meal.

One of those neurological effects is *cerebellar ataxia*, which is a loss of navigational ability and balance. As many as 22 percent of people with celiac disease suffer from it, and of all of the different types of ataxia diagnosed, 20 percent show abnormal blood markers for gluten. Of the people diagnosed with unexplained ataxia, 50 percent show abnormal blood markers for gluten. *(Hadjivassiliou et al. 2003)*

Unfortunately, ataxia is a progressive condition and usually results in limited mobility and motor function. Many people with ataxia also show impaired memory and cognitive function.

Wheat can also contribute to another disturbing neurological effect called *peripheral neuropathy*, which is a type of nerve damage that often affects the arms and legs. It's most often seen in diabetics, but is also diagnosed in people who are not diabetic and who are also not known to have celiac.

These conditions, of course, are in addition to the risks of dementia and Alzheimer's and the exacerbation of ADHD, schizophrenia, and autism that we've discussed in the previous chapter.

The Symptoms of Brain Function Impairment

The common symptoms of blood sugar crashing are probably familiar to you: fatigue, mental fogginess, impaired memory, and a lack of focus are just some of the neurological symptoms.

The symptoms of ataxia are harder to pin down, as many can also be attributed to other causes. However, common symptoms include loss of balance, frequent falls, and symptoms similar to early-onset Alzheimer's.

The symptoms of peripheral neuropathy are tingling or numbness in the hands, feet, arms, and legs. Often, people who exhibit signs of peripheral neuropathy are also diagnosed with type 2 diabetes.

The Wheat-Free Diet's Impact on Brain Function

Unfortunately, ataxia cannot be reversed once it's present, but eliminating wheat from the diet has been shown to stop its progression. Of course, it can also help to prevent the disorder.

As we've already discussed, eliminating wheat can help to reverse type 2 diabetes and prevent diseases such as peripheral neuropathy before they develop. Once diagnosed, however, this condition is not reversible. Like ataxia, it can be kept from growing more severe by eliminating wheat from the diet.

The symptoms of blood sugar crashing, such as fogginess, impaired memory, and a lack of focus, have been shown to disappear once the addiction to carbs is overcome—often within just a couple of weeks.

Insulin

We've already discussed the connection between wheat in the diet and impaired insulin response and secretion. Numerous studies have shown that the high blood glucose caused by eating wheat can be blamed for impaired insulin response or insulin resistance and that the storage of visceral fat that results exacerbates the problem.

The Symptoms of Insulin Resistance

Although increased abdominal fat can be a sign that you've become resistant to insulin, insulin resistance and metabolic syndrome don't have much in the way of visible symptoms. The National Diabetes Information Clearinghouse (NDIC), a service of the National Institute of Diabetes and Digestive and Kidney Diseases (NIDDK) and the National Institutes of Health (NIH), explains it this way:

> *Insulin resistance and prediabetes usually have no symptoms. People may have one or both conditions for several years without noticing anything. People with a severe form of insulin resistance may have dark patches of skin, usually on the back of the neck. Sometimes people have a dark ring around their neck. Other possible sites for dark patches include elbows, knees, knuckles, and armpits. This condition is called acanthosis nigricans.* **(NDIC 2008)**

The only way to determine if you are insulin resistant is to have your blood sugar tested.

The Wheat-Free Diet's Impact on Insulin Resistance

Insulin resistance or prediabetes has been shown in numerous studies to be reversible with reduced carbohydrate and sugar intake, including whole grains and whole-wheat products.

Eliminating wheat from your diet has many insulin-related benefits. Insulin balance and function return to normal as early as a few months after eliminating wheat. The visceral fat caused by insulin resistance is also known to be more readily utilized for energy than subcutaneous fat, which means that once your insulin levels are normalized, your body will start to use that stored visceral fat as energy. Not only will you lose visceral fat, but also excess abdominal fat.

The loss of visceral fat from going wheat-free will also help your affected organs, such as your liver and kidneys, to function more efficiently.

pH Balance

Our bodies are designed to operate at an optimum pH balance of 7.4. The pH balance is the balance of acidity and alkalinity in the blood. Even minute changes in pH balance can wreak havoc on your body. One of the most detrimental things for pH balance is a high-acid diet. The recent advent of "alkaline diets" and "pH diets" are answers to this problem. Foods can be classified as acidic, alkaline, or neutral. Wheat, surprisingly to most people, is highly acidic. In fact, wheat accounts for as much as 38 percent of the average American's acid intake. *(Davis 2011)*

The Connection Between Wheat and pH Balance

When the body is faced with a high acid intake, it tries to compensate by increasing alkalinity in the blood. Unfortunately, one of the chief ways it does this is by drawing calcium carbonate and calcium phosphate from the bones. This results in a loss of bone density and bone strength. A mild case of bone demineralization is known as *osteopenia,* while the more severe case is known as *osteoporosis.*

Interestingly, osteopenia and osteoporosis are virtually unknown in the skeletal remains of pre-agriculture, pre-wheat humans. It does begin to appear in skeletal remains of the last ten thousand years, which is when humans began harvesting, eating, and growing wheat. *(Frassetto et al. 2001)*

Symptoms of pH Imbalance

An acidic blood pH, or *acidosis*, can be hard to identify. Some of the common symptoms of early-stage acidosis include drowsiness and disorientation.

An acidic pH is more likely to be discovered because of bone fractures than it is because of any mild symptoms. These bone fractures aren't necessarily the more common types, such as breaking a leg when you fall from a bicycle. In advanced cases, even a sneeze can cause a break in the vertebrae of someone with long-term acidosis. *(Davis 2011)*

The Wheat-Free Diet's Impact on pH Balance

Obviously, removing one of the most acidic foods known, one that accounts for such a huge percentage of the average person's acid intake, is going to have a positive and dramatic impact on the body's pH balance.

Fortunately, blood pH corrects itself quickly, often in a matter of just a few weeks. While bone demineralization (osteopenia and osteoporosis) may have already occurred in advanced cases, further bone loss can be prevented, and there are medications that can help strengthen weakened bones.

Skin Health

There are several ways that wheat indirectly affects the health and appearance of your skin. The inflammation caused by wheat can produce everything from hives to a puffy appearance. However, wheat can damage your skin in many other ways.

The Connection Between Wheat and Skin Problems

One of the biggest impacts on skin comes in the form of acne. Many recent studies have shown that in cultures where wheat was not consumed, acne was virtually nonexistent. These cultures include the Inuit of Alaska, the Zulus of Africa, and the Kitavans of New Guinea. *(Cordain 2002)*

Even the Japanese Okinawans had virtually no acne among the population prior to the 1980s. However, when wheat became part of their diet, acne suddenly became a problem. The same is true of the Inuit. *(Miyagi et al. 2003)*

It's thought that the cause of the problem can once again be traced to insulin. Insulin stimulates the release of a hormone called *insulin-like growth factor 1*, or IGF-1, and IGF-1 then stimulates tissue growth in hair follicles and in the dermis layer of the skin, which is just beneath the skin's surface. Insulin and IGF-1 also promote the production of sebum, which is the oily, protective material created by the sebaceous glands. Too much sebum (which most people refer to as oily skin) leads to issues with acne. *(Cordain 2002)*

The Wheat-Free Diet's Impact on Skin Problems

The skin responds quite rapidly to changes in diet, including the elimination of wheat. Many people see clearer skin and fewer acne breakouts within a month of eliminating wheat from the diet, though it can take longer and there are other factors that influence sebum production.

However, the reduction of inflammation and the improvement of kidney function that result from eliminating wheat also have a positive effect on the skin. As visceral fat is lost, kidney function improves, and impurities that show up in the skin are reduced.

DID YOU KNOW? *Women with polycystic ovarian syndrome often have higher blood glucose and insulin production and are extremely prone to acne. When they take medications such as metformin to reduce insulin and glucose, they show a remarkable improvement in their skin. Young people who take medication for high blood sugar and excess insulin also see marked improvement.* (Davis 2011)

Weight

As we've discussed in previous chapters, a diet high in wheat products typically results in excess calories and weight. In addition, the hormone imbalance caused by eating wheat (specifically the hunger and stress hormones leptin, ghrelin, and cortisol) causes many people to overeat and to store more of what they eat as abdominal fat.

A diet high in carbohydrates is now widely accepted as being a recipe for weight gain and obesity as well as a host of other problems, such as type 2 diabetes.

The Symptoms of Obesity

Obviously, the chief symptoms of being overweight are a larger number on the scale and a larger clothing size. Many people who eat a low-carb diet take in the same number of calories as those on a high-carb diet, yet they maintain a healthy weight. This may be due in part to a faster metabolism or getting more exercise, but many nutritionists and researchers agree that excess carbs lead to excess weight, even when the daily caloric intake is the same as a low-carb diet. Our bodies simply don't need the excess carbs, so they store them as fat.

The Wheat-Free Diet's Impact on Weight

Numerous studies have shown that eliminating wheat products from the diet allows many people to lose weight. People with celiac are often underweight and malnourished when they're diagnosed and will often gain (much-needed and welcome) weight on a wheat-free diet because their bodies are able to absorb more nutrients. However, there are quite a few overweight and even obese people with celiac, and the weight-loss effect of going wheat-free has been studied extensively in these patients.

One study conducted by the Mayo Clinic with the University of Iowa followed 215 obese celiac patients upon their transition to a wheat-free diet. Those patients experienced an average weight loss of twenty-seven-and-a-half pounds during the first six months of living wheat-free. *(Murray et al. 2004)*

In another study published in 2010, obese participants were placed on a wheat-free diet. Within one year, the number of participants who were classified as obese was cut by an extraordinary 50 percent. *(Cheng et al. 2010)*

Wheat Allergies

Obviously, a wheat allergy is an intolerance or sensitivity to wheat. In this way, it differs from gluten sensitivity or celiac disease in that those conditions are an intolerance of the gluten in wheat, while wheat allergy is a reaction to the wheat itself, not the gluten. It is a food allergy, much like an allergy to peanuts or milk. Because of this difference, people with a wheat allergy are allowed to eat other gluten-containing grains such as rye, oats, and barley.

The Symptoms of Wheat Allergy

Many people with a wheat allergy first believe that they have celiac disease. This is understandable, since there are some shared symptoms between the two and they seem to be triggered by many of the same foods. The symptoms of wheat allergy are varied and can run the gamut from mild to severe. Common symptoms include swelling, itching, or irritation of the mouth or throat, hives, itchy rash or swelling of the skin, nasal congestion, itchy or watery eyes, breathing difficulties, digestive issues such as diarrhea, nausea, and cramps, and even in severe cases swelling of the throat.

The Wheat-Free Diet's Impact on Wheat Allergy

The elimination of wheat from the diet has an immediate positive impact on wheat allergy and its symptoms. Simple avoidance of the trigger is all it takes to eliminate allergic reactions. If you suspect you have a wheat allergy but eliminating wheat does not stop your symptoms, you should be tested for celiac disease, as many other grains contain gluten and your problem may be with gluten, not just wheat.

DID YOU KNOW? *Gluten is what gives dough its elasticity and helps it rise. Gluten can be separated from the dough by rinsing the dough repeatedly in water. Separated gluten is often used as a stabilizer in foods that don't normally contain wheat, such as some soy sauces and other condiments. Because the FDA doesn't require wheat to be listed as an ingredient when it's used in tiny amounts as a filler or stabilizer, this gluten is often referred to as "hidden gluten" and presents a real problem for people who are glucose intolerant or have celiac disease.*

Gluten Intolerance

Because very few wheat-based products are made with the gluten removed, wheat must be eliminated from the diet, along with other gluten-containing grasses such as barley and rye.

Gluten intolerance differs from celiac disease in a number of ways. There is no specific test that can be used to diagnose gluten intolerance, as there may be gluten antibodies present (as with celiac). However, celiac disease can be ruled out if there is no damage to the microvilli in the intestinal tract. (More on that in the next section.) The lack of damage to the microvilli, coupled with the patient's medical history and adverse symptoms when eating gluten, usually will lead the doctor to a diagnosis of gluten intolerance.

The Symptoms of Gluten Intolerance

Gluten intolerance may differ from celiac disease in many ways, but the two problems do share some of the same symptoms. Primarily, the symptoms of gluten intolerance are gastrointestinal and include gas, diarrhea, nausea, and bloating. Some people also suffer from frequent headaches and excessive tiredness.

The Wheat-Free Diet's Impact on Gluten Intolerance

As with wheat allergy, the elimination of wheat from the diet produces immediate results. With gluten intolerance, products made with barley, oats, and rye also have to be eliminated, as they also contain gluten.

Celiac Disease

The connection between wheat and celiac disease is clear and well documented. No one disputes the fact that celiac disease is directly connected to the consumption of wheat and other gluten-containing grains such as oats, barley, and rye.

In the simplest terms, celiac disease is an inability to process wheat that results in an inflammatory reaction. The immune system of celiac sufferers sees gluten as a foreign body and attacks it. The casualty of this reaction is the villi or microvilli of the small intestine.

The villi are microscopic fingerlike protuberances that line the small intestine. Their job is to absorb nutrients from foods as they pass by on their way to the large intestine, where whatever is leftover will be eliminated as waste.

With celiac disease, the villi become flattened and are unable to absorb the vitamins, minerals, fats, and other nutrients from food. These vital nutrients are passed right out of the body, and this eventually causes malnourishment (usually the first sign of celiac). Many people with celiac disease go misdiagnosed or undiagnosed for years before extreme weight loss and malnourishment alert a physician to the possibility of celiac.

Children are often diagnosed more easily than adults, as pediatricians keep a close eye on weight gain, growth, and development and can more easily see when a child isn't thriving as he should.

DID YOU KNOW? *The wheat genes most targeted for genetic modification are those found in the D-genome, which is the one most often blamed as the source of the gluten that triggers symptoms of celiac disease.*

The Symptoms of Celiac Disease

The symptoms of celiac disease are varied and can also differ in intensity from one person to another. The most common symptoms are abdominal swelling, constipation, bloating, diarrhea, fatty stools, gas, unexplained weight loss, fatigue, migraines, anemia, and nausea.

The Wheat-Free Diet's Impact on Celiac Disease

The positive impact of eliminating wheat and other gluten-containing grains cannot be overstated. It is only by eliminating gluten from the diet that people with celiac disease can find relief from its symptoms. In some cases, it's lifesaving, as malnourishment will continue if unchecked, resulting in eventual organ failure or death.

The time it takes for the villi to regenerate and begin to absorb nutrients properly will vary. Much depends on the severity of the disease and the length of time that it has gone untreated. However, eliminating gluten from the diet does eventually mean healing.

LIVING WHEAT-FREE

Embarking on a wheat-free lifestyle isn't as simple as eliminating pasta and cereals from your diet.

Wheat, gluten, and wheat proteins that are often called something other than wheat can be found in thousands of products. Many of these are in foods that you would never suspect contained wheat or gluten.

It's also important to understand the difference between wheat-free, gluten-free, grain-free, and any combination thereof and to decide which one you want to undertake. If you don't have celiac, you may want to be less vigilant than someone who does. If you have a wheat allergy, you may still want to eat oats, even though they produce much the same blood sugar/insulin response as wheat. If you have celiac or gluten intolerance, you'll want to eliminate all gluten-containing grains. These are the decisions that you'll need to make before you get started.

You'll also need to know how to go about the whole process, what to expect, and how to succeed in the transition. That's what this chapter is all about.

Wheat-Free, Gluten-Free, Grain-Free: What's the Difference?

The confusion about what a wheat-free diet means is understandable, but it's fairly easy to clear up. First, let's talk about grains other than wheat.

It's not necessary for you to give up all grains on the wheat-free diet. That's the Paleo diet, which eschews all grains because they are cultivated crops that humans didn't eat prior to about ten thousand years ago. There's certainly nothing wrong with the Paleo diet or the reasoning and research behind it, but the wheat-free diet doesn't mean eliminating all of the other grains.

That said, many grains, such as oats and rice, produce about the same blood sugar/insulin reaction as wheat, so these and other starchy grains, if you choose to eat them, should be eaten in moderate amounts. They should also be eaten with protein and fats to lower their overall glycemic load.

If you have gluten intolerance or celiac disease, then you'll need to eliminate not just wheat but all gluten-containing products and be especially careful of "hidden gluten." A list of many of the foods and other products that contain these hidden glutens can be found later in this chapter.

Those undertaking the wheat-free diet because it's a healthy choice, but who have no known intolerance or celiac risk, can afford to be a bit more relaxed. You may want to be vigilant about pastas, breads, cakes, and other foods that are high in wheat, but less so about hidden glutens and traces of gluten in things like condiments.

Regardless of how vigilant you are, you'll reap the rewards of a healthier, leaner body and a clearer mind.

Embracing the Wheat-Free Lifestyle

Going wheat-free can be a gradual process for those who don't have an urgent medical reason for eliminating wheat. If you fall into this category, don't overwhelm yourself thinking that every trace of wheat must be gone from your life by tomorrow morning. Making healthful lifestyle changes should be exciting and motivating, not stressful or overwhelming. If you decide to take up jogging for your health, you shouldn't expect to start by competing in a marathon. By the same token, you shouldn't expect to completely change all of your diet habits at once or without a few slips.

Make a plan to go wheat-free in steps that make sense for your health, your lifestyle, and your commitment. If your plan involves taking several weeks to eliminate all wheat, that's fine. Start with the big wheat culprits and work your way down, or eliminate the least healthful foods in your diet and end by eliminating the supposedly healthful ones. Find your comfort level and don't worry about following anything to the letter.

Try to focus on the benefits of going wheat-free, rather than on the dangers of the wheat-filled diet you've been eating. Focusing on your increased energy, lost weight, healthier digestive system, and clearer skin is a lot more motivating and a lot less stressful than worrying about every single thing you eat.

Try also to celebrate each positive step that you do take and each victory over your old way of eating, no matter how small. If you finally manage to swap out your beloved breakfast cereal for a more healthful, flax-seed porridge, give yourself your proper due.

In the end, adopting a wheat-free diet is all about achieving better health and greater happiness. Focus on those goals more than you focus on what you're missing and you'll be able to embrace the wheat-free lifestyle with a smile.

What to Eat

The purpose of the wheat-free diet is not only to eliminate most if not all of the wheat and gluten in your diet, but also to eat a low-carb, low-glycemic diet in order to correct the blood sugar/insulin cycle caused by your former, wheat-filled diet.

There's no need to get into an exhaustive list of which foods you can eat. That purpose will be better served by listing the foods you cannot eat. However, there are some guidelines that you can follow regarding the foods you want to include in your diet.

For the most part, the best way to create your wheat-free, low-glycemic diet is to focus on whole foods. This means getting the majority of your daily foods from fresh produce, fresh meats and seafood, nuts, seeds, healthful fats, and a few grains in moderation. With whole foods, you don't have to read labels or memorize and decipher code words for wheat and gluten, trying to determine if gluten or wheat products are lurking in your soup. Prepare your own from scratch and you'll know exactly what's in it.

Let's take a look at the different categories of foods and which varieties of these foods you should be eating.

Fruits

Fruits also provide essential nutrients and are a delicious food that can satisfy a sweet tooth just as easily as a candy bar . . . once you've retrained your palate. As with vegetables, you need to watch the glycemic index of these important foods.

These fruits all have a glycemic index of 60 or below and should be the mainstays of your fruit supplies:

- Apples
- Apricots
- Avocadoes
- Bananas
- Blackberries
- Cantaloupe
- Cherries
- Cranberries
- Grapefruit
- Guavas

- Kiwis
- Lemons
- Limes
- Oranges
- Papayas
- Peaches
- Plums
- Raspberries
- Rhubarb
- Strawberries
- Tangerines
- Tomatoes

These fruits have a glycemic index of over 60 and should be enjoyed less frequently or eliminated from your diet:

- Any dried fruit
- Blueberries
- Figs
- Grapes
- Kumquats
- Loganberries
- Mangoes
- Mulberries
- Pears
- Pineapples
- Pomegranates

Vegetables

Vegetables are a wonderful and essential part of a healthful diet. Corn and white potatoes are the only vegetables that you really shouldn't eat, as they are actually starches that convert very quickly to sugar. That said, you should focus most of your attention on those vegetables that have a lower glycemic index.

These vegetables all have a glycemic index of less than 20 and should be your go-to veggies:

- Asparagus
- Bean sprouts
- Beet greens
- Broccoli
- Cabbages
- Cauliflowers
- Celery
- Cucumbers
- Endive
- Lettuces
- Mustard greens
- Radishes
- Spinach
- Swiss chard
- Watercress

These vegetables have a glycemic index of 60 or less and can also be eaten frequently:

- Beets
- Brussels sprouts
- Chives
- Collards

- Dandelion leaves
- Eggplants
- Kale
- Kohlrabi
- Leeks
- Okra
- Onions
- Parsley
- Peas
- Peppers
- Pimento peppers
- Pumpkins
- Rutabagas
- String beans
- Turnips

The following vegetables have a glycemic index over 60 and should be eaten rarely or reserved as occasional treats:

- Artichokes
- Carrots
- Dried beans
- Lima beans
- Oyster plants
- Parsnips
- Squashes
- Sweet potatoes
- Yams

Dairy Products

The sugars that naturally occur in cow's milk or goat's milk are more quickly converted to glucose than you would like. Try swapping them out with almond or coconut milk in your cereal, smoothies, and cooking, and use the animal-based milks only on special occasions.

Because some aged cheeses are fermented with wheat, you want to eliminate them from your diet. These include bleu, Roquefort, Gorgonzola, and some cottage cheese. Cheeses such as mozzarella, Swiss, and goat cheese are fine.

When you consume dairy products, coupling them with protein or fiber lowers their glycemic load. An excellent example is Greek yogurt, which packs twice the protein of regular yogurt and is an excellent food to include in your diet. Fruity-syrupy yogurts are to be avoided, as are those made with artificial sweeteners such as aspartame.

Fish, Seafood, and Meats

You can basically enjoy any meat or seafood on the wheat-free diet, with the exception of cured and processed meats, such as some bacon, hot dogs, cold cuts, sausage, and smoked fish. These almost always contain added sugar, and often contain wheat-based fillers and stabilizers.

Grains

Grains should be kept to a fairly low profile in your diet. As discussed earlier, how much you restrict grains other than wheat will depend partly on whether you have celiac disease or gluten intolerance, but it's recommended that you eliminate most grains or at least keep them to a minimum.

One wonderful food to stand in for the wheat-based pasta you think you'll miss is shirataki noodles. Used for centuries in China and Japan, shirataki noodles, also sold as "Miracle Noodles," are made entirely from non-digestible plant fiber. They have no carbs and no calories. They look and feel like regular pasta and are available in many varieties. You can find them online and in many health food stores.

Healthful Fats

Fat is an essential component of a healthful diet, and you should get enough of it in your diet. Olive oil, olives, canola oil, coconut oil, nuts, cold-water fish, and avocadoes are all good sources.

Nuts and Seeds

Nuts and seeds are a great source of fiber, protein, and healthful fats. You should, of course, eat those that have no added sugar, and you're better off with unsalted nuts (reserve the salted nuts for treat time).

Nut and seed flours are actually a great alternative to wheat and other flours. Ground flax seed makes a great hot cereal and can even be used in your baking. You can find it in health food stores, online at a gluten-free retailer, or sometimes even in your supermarket (usually in the organic section).

The only caveat here is to pass up peanuts and soy nuts. They're actually legumes and have the same bad effect on blood sugar as starches and wheat.

What to Avoid

The following is a fairly exhaustive list of foods containing wheat, gluten, and wheat by-products that should be eliminated from your diet, courtesy of Dr. William Davis:

Additives, Fillers, Colorings, and Stabilizers

Artificial colors, artificial flavors, caramel coloring, caramel flavoring, Dextri-Maltose, emulsifiers, maltodextrin, modified food starch, stabilizers, and textured vegetable protein.

Beverages

Ales, beers, and lagers (though there are some gluten-free varieties); Bloody Mary mix; flavored coffees and herbal teas made with wheat, barley, or malt; malt liquor; flavored vodkas distilled from wheat; wine coolers containing barley malt; whisky distilled from wheat or barley.

Breakfast Cereals

Any cereal obviously made from wheat, plus bran cereals, corn flakes, granola cereals, muesli, oat cereals, popped-corn cereals, and puffed-rice cereals.

Energy, Protein, and "Health" Bars

Clif Bars, Gatorade Pre-Game Fuel Nutrition bars, GNC Pro Performance bars, Kashi GOLEAN bars, PowerBars, and Slim-Fast bars.

Hot Cereals

Cream of Wheat, farina, Malt-O-Meal, instant oatmeal, and oat bran.

Prepared Soups

Bisques, broths, bouillon, canned soups, soup mixes, soup stocks, and soup bases.

Seasonings

Curry powder, seasoning mixes, and taco seasoning.

Sauces, Condiments, and Dressings*

*Some of these are available in gluten-free versions.

Gravies thickened with wheat flour, ketchup, malt syrup, malt vinegar, marinades, miso, mustards containing wheat, salad dressings, soy sauce, and teriyaki sauce.

Sweeteners

Barley malt, barley extract, dextrin and maltodextrin, malt, malt syrup, and malt flavoring.

Sweets and Snacks**

**Other than obvious wheat-based foods.

Cake frosting, candy bars, chewing gum (wheat-based powdered coating), Chex mixes, corn chips, dried fruit (lightly coated with flour), dry-roasted peanuts, fruit fillings with thickeners, jelly beans (not including Jelly Belly beans and Starburst candies), granola bars, some ice cream (cookies and cream, Oreo Cookie, cookie dough, cheesecake, chocolate malt), ice cream cones, licorice, nut bars, pies, potato chips (including Pringles), tiramisu, tortilla chips, and flavored trail mixes.

Possible Problematic Non-Food Items✳✳✳

✳✳✳Read labels carefully or speak to the manufacturer if you have celiac disease, wheat allergy, or gluten intolerance.

Envelopes, glue, paste, Play-Doh, stickers, labels, lip gloss, lip balms, lipstick, and stamps.

Alternative Ingredients

There are many good wheat-free, gluten-free versions of many of these foods, but you need to be careful about which ones you use. Many gluten-free products still contain wheat, and many wheat-free products still contain gluten. Also, many gluten-free flours are made of starches such as potato starch that are just as hard on your blood sugar as white flour. For condiments, sauces, and the like, read the labels carefully. For baked goods, snacks, and treats, it's much better to make your own.

A Word about Artificial Sweeteners

Artificial sweeteners are extremely unhealthful and should be avoided. Replace sugar and other sweeteners with Truvia or stevia and consult the label or recipes for the correct equivalent to use.

TRANSITIONING INTO
THE WHEAT-FREE DIET

Like all lifestyle changes, transitioning to a wheat-free diet requires some planning and forethought.

Every success is measured in steps, and there are several you can take to make your adoption of a wheat-free lifestyle as successful as possible, while still enjoying delicious foods and a happy social life. And remember, unless you have celiac disease or a wheat allergy, this doesn't have to happen all at once.

The most important things you can do to make the transition successfully are to prepare your home and family, get your attitude and mindset right, know what to expect from the transitional phase, and keep your eyes on your goal: a more healthful, happier life.

10 Tips for a Successful Transition

1.   *Prepare your friends and family for a change.*
     Let your family, friends, and coworkers know that you're making the change to a wheat-free diet. Not only do you need their emotional support, but you also need to help them help you. Let them know that you may not be able to go out for the same foods, that you need

to steer clear of the Friday morning doughnut ritual, or anything else that can help them avoid tripping you up or making you feel awkward.

If you have a spouse or children at home who will not be going wheat-free, you'll need to let them know what you're doing and why, how important it is to you, and what to expect.

2. **Prepare your kitchen.**

    This is especially important if you have celiac disease or gluten intolerance. Any foods containing wheat or gluten need to be removed from your home or (if you have other family at home) put in a completely separate area. With these conditions, even having your food or utensils come into contact with those that contain or have touched wheat/gluten can be harmful.

    If you don't have gluten intolerance or celiac disease, you still want to remove all forbidden foods from the kitchen. Donate them to friends or to a local charity or shelter. Then purchase the supplies that you do need from the list of foods in Chapter 4.

    You don't need any special tools or utensils to eat wheat-free, but there are some that can be great to have. A spice grinder or food processor can help you to make your own flours out of nuts and seeds. A stand mixer can also be a handy tool if you like to bake. Using a mixer will help you incorporate more air and to mix heavier nut and seed meals better than you can by hand.

3. **Get your mindset right.**

    Focus on the good you're doing, not the "good" things you think you're giving up. Believe it or not, there are wonderful wheat- and gluten-free recipes for some of your favorite treats—many of them in Chapter 6!

Understand and expect that the first few weeks will be the most difficult, but that the way you look and feel as you progress will more than make up for the time you spend withdrawing from and craving wheat.

4. *Be your own biggest supporter.*
    More likely than not, at some point in your transition, you're going to have a brownie, a slice of pizza, or a beer. That's why it's called a transition, not a transformation. Even when you slip, remind yourself that it's a very tiny step backward on the road to great health. Give yourself credit for making the commitment, instead of beating yourself up for making a mistake. That can lead to only frustration, loss of motivation, and a doughnut.

5. *Give yourself free reign on the allowed foods.*
    Even if one of your goals is to lose weight, don't try to cut calories or stick to a rigid calorie allowance as you're transitioning to a wheat-free lifestyle. As I discussed previously, most people will lose weight on the wheat-free diet without counting calories. Give your body a chance to adapt and to correct the imbalances in your hormones and metabolism. This can take as long as a couple of months or even six months. You most likely will be losing weight during this time, especially stored fat. Once your body has made its adjustments, if you still want to lose weight, you can look at your caloric intake. Better yet, exercise (if you aren't already).

6. *Focus more on discovering new foods than replicating old ones.*
    While it's perfectly all right to go in search of the perfect gluten-free/wheat-free brownie recipe, try not to obsess over replacing your old favorite treats with revamped versions. It can make your focus too centered on what you're missing, rather than on what you're gaining. Instead, discover new foods that you've never tried and new cuisines that you haven't sampled. Try one new fruit or

vegetable every week and start taste-testing unfamiliar types of fish or nuts. Make this time an adventure of discovery rather than a quest for what you think is lost.

7. **Cut back on food-centered activities if you need to.**
Food is very much a part of our culture and our social lives. Parties, happy hour, holidays, picnics, and fellowship are centered on food. There's no reason you can't still enjoy all of these things, but if you find it hard in the beginning, come up with ways to be social without food being the center of things. Meet friends for a glass of wine rather than doughnuts or dinner. Go for a hike instead of a picnic. Go to a bowling alley instead of a bar.

Think of things you can do with your friends and family that don't present so much of a problem for you. It'll get easier to navigate food and social occasions as you progress through the diet, and in the meantime, you may even have more fun.

8. **Get moving.**
There will be cravings and withdrawal from wheat in the beginning. Just like with quitting smoking, sometimes the best way to work through a craving is to work it out. When the going gets tough, the tough go walking, biking, swimming, or dancing. Not only will it help you take your mind off the craving until it passes, but it will also get those endorphins involved in calming your nerves.

9. **Find a buddy.**
See if you can find someone to go on the diet with you. If you don't have a friend or relative to buddy up with, look online at one of the many diet support forums. Online companionship, support, and accountability can be as valuable as buddying up with someone you know.

10. **Remember that this too shall pass.**

The transitional phase doesn't last forever. Most people report that they experience fewer cravings and withdrawal symptoms (such as fatigue, crankiness, and hunger) within just a week. And with some practice, the confusion about foods, products, and labels will go away just as quickly. You'll learn how to make brownies and you'll be asked to bring them to the next party or family get-together. Like starting at a new school, you'll quickly adjust to and learn to love your new lifestyle.

Wheat Withdrawal and How to Survive It

First the good news: Only about 30 percent of people experience symptoms of wheat withdrawal.

And those who do report that most, if not all, of their symptoms are gone within a week. Dr. Davis reported that he hadn't seen any cases of wheat withdrawal last more than four weeks. *(Davis 2011)*

Withdrawal symptoms usually take the form of listlessness, a feeling of sadness or low morale, fatigue, mental fogginess, and irritability. One interesting withdrawal symptom is the lack of capacity for exercise. It's very short-lived and a few days away from the gym won't hurt you.

The people who experience symptoms of withdrawal most are those who were knowingly addicted to carbs. They have the toughest transition, although it generally lasts only a week or two. If you think you're one of those people, you may want to try to schedule your first few days on the diet to coincide with a long weekend or even take a few vacation days. This will relieve you of the stress and complication of trying to look happy and be nice.

You may also try scheduling some one-on-one time with a close friend who can take your changing moods. Plan to do something fun but undemanding, even if that's just playing board games or window shopping.

Most importantly, remember that these withdrawal symptoms, if you are one of the 30 percent who experience them, will be over before you know it.

Wheat-Free Diet Seven-Day Meal Plan

One of the big concerns that many people have when deciding to make the transition to a wheat-free diet is meal planning. They worry that it will be too time-consuming, confusing, and/or boring.

While there will be some label reading and maybe some recipe gathering and testing, planning your meals really isn't that complicated. The big task is in getting used to replacing old standby starches and flour-based foods with healthier sides, snacks, or entrees. And you'll have that down in just a week or two.

Learning how to read labels does take some time, but you'll soon know the hidden wheat code words by heart and also know which prepared foods you need to forgo and which ones have good gluten-free/wheat-free versions.

As far as boredom, many people find that once they kick their wheat addiction and their almost careless food choices, they really begin to enjoy the huge variety of foods that are available that they may not have taken time to discover before.

Following are a week's worth of menu plans that can help you to get an idea of how you'll be eating. If you feel like it would be easier for you, you can follow them to the letter or simply use them as a guide.

(For dishes marked with an asterisk (*), you can find the recipes in Chapter 6.)

DAY 1

Breakfast
Scrambled eggs
Half of a cantaloupe
Sliced chicken breast

Snack
Black Bean Hummus Dip*
Celery

Lunch
Grilled chicken salad
Apple slices

Dinner
Pecan-Crusted Flounder*
Sautéed kale
Cucumber and pepper salad

Dessert
No-Flour Rich Chocolate Cake*

DAY 2

Breakfast
Mushroom and Pesto Omelet*
Sliced pear

Snack
Walnuts and sliced apple

Lunch
Simply Good Chicken Noodle Soup*
Romaine and mushroom salad

Dinner
Pork Loin with Roasted Sweet Potato Strips*
Steamed spinach

Dessert
Fresh apricot

DAY 3

Breakfast
Hearty Hot Flax Cereal*
Fresh plum

Snack
Vanilla Greek yogurt

Lunch
Beef vegetable soup
Veggie lettuce wrap

Dinner
Orange and Ginger Flank Steak Stir-Fry*

Dessert
Pecan-Apple Tart*

DAY 4

Breakfast
Morning Latte Smoothie*

Snack
Sliced apples with almond butter

Lunch
Roast beef au jus
Baked squash
Green salad

Dinner
Garlic and Herb Roasted Chicken*
Roasted asparagus
Green leafy salad

Dessert
Very Berry Dessert*

DAY 5

Breakfast
Greek yogurt with apples and walnuts

Snack
Spinach and Orange Salad with Sesame-Lime Dressing*

Lunch
Philly Lettuce Wraps*
Sliced avocado

Dinner
Grilled fish
Roasted Brussels sprouts

Dessert
Gluten-free ice cream

DAY 6

Breakfast
Quinoa Breakfast Parfait*

Snack
Cantaloupe chunks with cottage cheese

Lunch
Vegetable soup
Chicken drumstick
Fresh peach

Dinner
Shirataki Shrimp Scampi*
Green salad

Dessert
Baked apple

DAY 7

Breakfast
Sweet and Spicy Pumpkin Bread*
Soft-boiled eggs
Apple slices

Snack
Walnuts

Lunch
Creamy Tomato Soup*
Avocado, goat cheese, and onion salad

Dinner
Dilly-Orange Sole Steamed in Foil*
Sautéed Swiss chard with red peppers

Dessert
Gluten-free brownie

WHEAT-FREE RECIPES

Snacks and Appetizers

Smoked Salmon-Stuffed Tomatoes

This classic combination of salmon, cream cheese, and tomato makes a great dish that's versatile, too—serve it for lunch or at your next dinner party.

- 6 small plum tomatoes
- 4 ounces low-fat cream cheese
- 1 teaspoon Dijon mustard
- 2 teaspoons fresh dill, minced, plus additional dill for garnish, if desired
- ½ teaspoon freshly ground black pepper
- 8 ounces smoked salmon, chopped
- ¼ cup celery, finely chopped

Halve the plum tomatoes and use a melon baller or teaspoon to scrape the flesh onto a cutting board. Chop well and place in a medium mixing bowl.

Add the cream cheese, Dijon mustard, dill, and black pepper, and mix well.

Gently stir in the salmon and celery, and stir just until blended.

Using a teaspoon, divide the filling among the 12 tomato halves, leaving it piled high. Garnish with fresh dill if desired.

Makes 1 dozen.

Black Bean Hummus Dip

Hummus is traditionally prepared only with garbanzo beans, but the addition of black beans makes this hummus dip especially creamy. It keeps well in the refrigerator and makes a good snack for taking to work or school.

- ½ cup canned black beans, well drained
- ½ cup canned garbanzo beans, well drained
- ¼ cup tahini
- 2 cloves fresh garlic, crushed
- 4 tablespoons lemon juice
- ½ teaspoon salt
- 1 teaspoon olive oil

Combine black beans, garbanzo beans, tahini, garlic, lemon juice, and salt in a blender and mix until fairly smooth. Spoon into a serving dish, and drizzle with olive oil.

Serve with fresh vegetables, such as celery, cherry tomatoes, carrots, and red peppers.

Makes about 1½ cups.

Mediterranean Salad

This quick salad makes an appetizing start to an Italian meal or even a light lunch on a warm day. It's best made one day ahead, giving the flavors time to develop. If you choose to prepare it in advance, wait to add the Parmesan until ready to serve.

For the dressing:
- ¼ cup light olive oil
- ¼ cup balsamic vinegar
- 1 clove fresh garlic, crushed
- ½ teaspoon salt
- ½ teaspoon pepper

For the salad:
- 1 (10-ounce) can artichoke hearts, well drained and roughly chopped
- ½ cup cherry tomatoes, sliced
- ½ sweet white onion, thinly sliced
- ½ cup part-skim mozzarella, chopped into ½-inch cubes
- 2 teaspoons fresh basil, chopped
- 1 tablespoon freshly shaved Parmesan cheese

In a food processor, combine all of the dressing ingredients, and blend on medium-high speed until smooth. Taste for seasoning, and add salt and/or pepper if needed.

In a shallow casserole or baking dish, combine the artichoke hearts, tomatoes, onion, mozzarella, and basil, and stir well. Pour dressing over all, stir to mix well, and refrigerate for a minimum of 4 hours.

To serve, top with freshly shaved Parmesan.

Makes 4 servings.

Mushroom-Stuffed Mushrooms

Portobello mushrooms have a meaty taste and texture that can easily stand in for a beef entrée if you'd like a vegetarian meal. Otherwise, this dish makes a wonderfully earthy appetizer.

- 4 large whole portobello mushroom caps
- 2 tablespoons olive oil, divided
- 1½ teaspoons salt, divided
- ½ pound white button mushrooms, chopped
- 1 clove fresh garlic, chopped
- ¼ cup white onion, chopped fine
- 1 teaspoon paprika
- ½ teaspoon freshly ground black pepper
- ½ cup shredded Swiss cheese

Using your hands, rub 1 tablespoon olive oil onto the outsides of the portobello mushroom caps. Sprinkle with about ½ teaspoon salt, and place right-side up in a large, heavy skillet.

Cook uncovered over medium heat for 5 to 7 minutes without turning, then remove to a baking dish.

Preheat oven to 375 degrees.

Add a second tablespoon of olive oil to the same skillet and reduce heat to medium-low. Add chopped mushrooms, garlic, and onion. Add remaining teaspoon salt, paprika, and pepper, stirring well to blend.

Cook over low heat, stirring frequently for 5 minutes, and remove to a small bowl.

Add shredded Swiss cheese, stirring well, then divide the filling between the 4 portobello caps.

Bake for 8 to 10 minutes or until filling is browned and bubbly.

Makes 2-4 servings.

Spicy Crab and Cucumber Canapés

The cool sweetness of fresh cucumber is a great foil for this slightly spicy crab dip. This dish makes a terrific appetizer or light lunch.

- 2 medium cucumbers
- 1 teaspoon salt, divided
- 8 ounces imitation crab meat, flaked-style
- 1 red bell pepper, finely chopped
- 1 stalk celery, finely sliced
- 2 tablespoons light mayonnaise
- ½ teaspoon garlic powder
- ½ teaspoon chili powder
- ½ teaspoon cumin
- ½ teaspoon freshly ground black pepper
- Fresh dill to garnish

Cut the ends from both cucumbers, and use the tines of a fork to score the skins all the way around.

Slice the cucumbers ¼ inch thick, sprinkle with about ½ teaspoon salt, and set aside.

Using your hands, shred the imitation crab into a medium mixing bowl. Add the bell pepper and celery.

In a small bowl, combine the mayonnaise, remaining salt, garlic powder, chili powder, cumin, and black pepper, and mix well. Add to crab mixture, and stir until blended. Taste for seasoning, and add remaining salt and additional pepper if desired.

Spread 1 tablespoon of the crab mixture onto each cucumber slice, and garnish with dill if desired. Cover and chill for 1 hour before serving.

Makes about 24 pieces or 6 servings.

Seafood-Stuffed Shells

This creamy seafood dish is a variation on a popular recipe for mussels. If you prefer to serve this as a dip, simply place filling into a shallow gratin dish before broiling, rather than spooning into the shells.

- ½ cup dry white wine
- 1 teaspoon sea salt
- 12 large live clams
- ½ pound precooked shrimp, chopped
- ¼ cup mayonnaise
- ¼ cup light cream cheese
- 8-10 drops of Tabasco sauce (to taste)
- 1 teaspoon Worcestershire sauce
- ¼ cup fresh parsley, chopped

In a large heavy pot, combine 2 cups water, white wine, and salt. Bring to a boil and add clams. Cover and cook about 5 to 7 minutes or until clams have opened. Remove from pot and set aside to cool.

Break cooled clam shells in half, place clams on a cutting board, and place shells in a 9 x 13-inch baking dish. Chop clams and put into a medium mixing bowl. Add shrimp and stir well.

In a blender or food processor, combine mayonnaise, cream cheese, Tabasco sauce, Worcestershire, and fresh parsley, and blend just until combined.

Add cheese mixture to the clams and shrimp, and stir to mix well.

Preheat broiler.

Spoon mixture into clam shells, and broil for 3 to 4 minutes, just until bubbly.

Makes 4 servings.

Spinach and Orange Salad with Sesame-Lime Dressing

Even in the cold of winter, this fresh, citrusy salad will bring the taste of summer home. The dressing is a variation of a famous honey-lime dressing from Disney's 'Ohana Resort. Be sure to use regular lime juice, not Key lime. The dressing keeps very well for up to a month, so make extra to keep on hand in the fridge.

For the dressing:

- ½ cup cider vinegar
- ¼ cup lime juice
- ½ teaspoon Dijon mustard
- ¼ cup sweet white onion, chopped
- 2 teaspoons toasted sesame seeds
- 1 teaspoon liquid stevia extract
- 1 cup canola oil

For the salad:

- 2 cups fresh spinach leaves
- ½ red bell pepper, chopped
- ½ cup white button mushrooms, sliced
- 2 large navel oranges, peeled and sectioned, membrane removed

In a blender, mix the vinegar, lime juice, mustard, onion, sesame seeds, and stevia. Blend until smooth. Slowly pour canola oil into blender while blending on low speed, and blend for 1 minute until creamy.

In a salad bowl, combine spinach, peppers, mushrooms, and oranges, and toss well.

Pour dressing over all and toss again.

Makes 2 servings.

Crispy Kale Chips

Kale is loaded with vitamins and minerals and is a popular side dish similar to spinach. When dried in the oven, it also makes one of the tastiest and most addictive snacks you'll ever try. After one batch of these, you won't be tempted by greasy potato chips.

- 2 bunches fresh kale, washed and dried
- 4 tablespoons extra-virgin olive oil
- 1 teaspoon salt

Preheat oven to 250 degrees.

Make sure the kale is completely dry, then remove all ribs and rip each leaf in half, placing the torn leaves in a large salad or mixing bowl.

Toss the kale with olive oil, using your hands to distribute the oil evenly.

Spread the kale onto a large baking sheet and sprinkle with salt.

Bake in the center of the oven for 15 minutes. Use tongs to turn each leaf, and return to the oven for another 10 minutes.

Serve immediately.

Makes 6 servings.

Pear and Prosciutto Packets

Prosciutto is a rare treat for many people, and this very simple recipe is a delicious way to make the most of the occasion. It's also a nice change from the traditional prosciutto and melon.

- 3 pears, peeled and cut into chunks
- 1/3 cup lime juice
- 1/2 pound prosciutto
- 5 ounces Brie
- 1/2 teaspoon freshly ground pepper

In a medium mixing bowl, toss the pear chunks in the lime juice, coating well. Drain off any excess juice.

Cut prosciutto slices about 2- to 2½-inches long and set aside.

Place a chunk of pear about ⅓ of the way up a slice of prosciutto, smear with just enough brie to cover the top of the pear, and sprinkle with freshly ground pepper.

Roll the close end of the prosciutto up over the pear and continue rolling the pear to the end. Fasten with a toothpick. Continue with the rest of the pears.

Chill for 1 hour and arrange on a platter to serve.

Makes about 18 pieces.

Spicy Roasted Nuts

These spicy, crunchy snacks are a great way to start a party or satisfy the urge for something salty. They keep well in an airtight container, so pack some to take to work. The protein, fiber, and healthy fats they contain will keep you from raiding the vending machine.

- 1 cup shelled walnut halves
- 1 cup unsalted roasted almonds
- 1 cup shelled sunflower seeds
- 1 teaspoon olive oil
- 1 teaspoon salt
- 1 teaspoon cumin
- ½ teaspoon cayenne pepper

In a large bowl, coat the walnuts, almonds, and sunflower seeds with olive oil, tossing well.

Add the salt, cumin, and cayenne pepper, and toss well again.

Heat a heavy skillet over medium heat, and add the nut mixture. Cook, stirring well, for 10 minutes.

Cool to room temperature before placing in a zippered freezer bag or airtight container.

Makes about 6 servings.

Breakfast

Mushroom and Pesto Omelet

Some people think omelets are a bit complicated, but they're actually a very quick meal to prepare and a great way to pack plenty of nutrients into one dish. This recipe uses prepared pesto to create a delicious meal that will carry you through the morning.

- 3 large eggs
- 1 teaspoon water
- 1 teaspoon extra-virgin olive oil
- 1 tablespoon prepared pesto
- ¼ cup tomato, diced
- ¼ cup fresh mushrooms, sliced
- Salt and pepper to taste

In a small mixing bowl, whisk together the eggs and water.

Heat a medium skillet over medium-high heat and add the olive oil, turning the pan to coat.

Pour in the eggs, and tilt the pan to spread the eggs evenly over the bottom. Cook until the eggs are mostly dry in the center, using a spatula to occasionally pull the edges in and allow uncooked egg to run to the edges of the pan and cook.

Flip the omelet, and reduce heat to medium-low.

Spread the pesto over half of the eggs, and add tomatoes and mushrooms. Fold the bare half of the eggs over the other to form the omelet, cook for 1 minute, and slide onto a plate.

Add salt and pepper to taste and serve.

Makes 1 serving.

Hearty Hot Flax Cereal

Flax seed is loaded with fiber, omega-3 fats, protein, and other essential nutrients. You can buy ground flax seed in the organic section of your supermarket or in your local health food store. It makes a wonderfully nutty, hot cereal and is especially hearty in this quick recipe.

- ½ cup plus 1 tablespoon unflavored almond milk, divided
- ¼ teaspoon salt
- ½ cup ground flax seed
- ¼ cup walnut halves, roughly chopped
- 2 tablespoons dried cranberries
- ½ teaspoon Stevia In The Raw
- ½ medium banana, sliced

In a medium saucepan, heat ½ cup unflavored almond milk and salt on medium heat, just until it reaches a simmer.

Add the flax seed, walnuts, cranberries, and stevia, and cook, stirring constantly, for 3 minutes.

To serve, ladle into a deep bowl, and top with bananas and 1 tablespoon unflavored almond milk.

Makes 1 serving.

Morning Latte Smoothie

That coffee drink you pick up on the way to work gets expensive and offers little in the way of nutrition. This recipe is delicious, quick to make, and fits right into a travel mug. Allow your espresso to cool to room temperature while you get ready—this shake will take just thirty seconds to whip up on your way out the door.

- ¾ cup vanilla-flavored almond milk
- 1 or 2 shots brewed espresso, cooled to room temperature
- ½ teaspoon liquid stevia extract, or to taste
- ½ teaspoon cinnamon
- 6-8 ice cubes

In a blender, combine almond milk, espresso, stevia, and cinnamon, and blend on high for about 15 seconds.

Add ice cubes and blend until thick and smooth. Pour into a glass or travel mug to serve.

If you prefer your latte hot, omit the ice and add an additional ¼ cup vanilla-flavored almond milk. In this case, there's no need to cool the espresso.

Makes 1 serving.

Quinoa Breakfast Parfait

Cereals and granolas are often some of the hardest foods for people to give up. This nutty, fruity breakfast parfait is loaded not only with flavor and texture, but a healthy dose of fiber and protein. It'll keep you going all morning, and you'll never miss a thing.

- 1 cup cooked quinoa, prepared according to package directions
- 1 ripe Bartlett or Bosc pear, peeled, cored, and cut into chunks
- 1 cup vanilla-flavored Greek yogurt
- ½ cup black walnut pieces
- 2 teaspoons sugar-free maple syrup (made with stevia extract)

Divide quinoa between 2 dessert dishes or bowls. Top each with half the pear.

Add ½ cup vanilla-flavored Greek yogurt to each dish, and sprinkle each serving with ¼ cup walnut pieces.

To serve, drizzle each serving with sugar-free maple syrup.

Makes 2 servings.

Sweet and Spicy Pumpkin Bread

This extremely dense and moist pumpkin bread is a delicious way to start your day and also makes a tasty snack. It will keep very well for up to a week if wrapped in plastic and stored in an airtight container.

- ¾ cup plain canned pumpkin
- ¼ cup tahini
- 1 tablespoon canola oil
- 3 large eggs, beaten
- 1 teaspoon liquid stevia extract
- ¼ cup almond meal
- ¼ cup arrowroot powder

- 1 teaspoon salt
- 1 teaspoon cinnamon
- ½ teaspoon nutmeg
- ½ teaspoon ground ginger
- ½ teaspoon baking powder
- ¼ teaspoon baking soda
- ½ cup chopped walnuts

Preheat oven to 325 degrees and grease a 9 x 4-inch loaf pan.

In a large bowl, combine pumpkin, tahini, stevia, and canola oil until well blended. Add eggs and beat with a hand mixer on low setting until eggs are well incorporated. Set aside.

In a separate large bowl, combine almond meal, arrowroot, salt, cinnamon, nutmeg, ginger, baking powder, and baking soda. Stir with a whisk or wooden spoon until thoroughly blended. Add in walnuts and again mix well.

Slowly add dry ingredients to wet ingredients, using hand mixer on low speed to incorporate all of the dry ingredients. Be sure to scrape any dry ingredients from the side of the bowl while mixing.

Continue to mix until all dry ingredients are incorporated, then pour batter into prepared loaf pan.

Bake on the center rack of the oven for 50 minutes or until a toothpick inserted in the center comes out clean.

Allow to cool in the loaf pan for 15 minutes before turning out onto a wire rack to cool completely.

Serve as is or toast slices in a regular or toaster oven, and spread with whipped cream cheese.

Makes about 10 servings.

Savory Morning Hash

This is a wonderful breakfast dish for lazy weekend mornings, especially when the weather gets cool. Use fresh, uncured sausage if possible, as the cured variety usually contains far too much sugar and preservatives.

- 1 pound turkey sausage, casings removed
- ½ teaspoon rosemary
- ½ teaspoon ground sage
- 2 teaspoons olive oil, divided
- 4 large eggs

- 2 Granny Smith or Gala apples, peeled, cored, and cut into 1-inch pieces
- ½ cup sweet white onion, diced
- Salt and freshly ground black pepper to taste

Crumble sausage into a medium mixing bowl, and stir in rosemary and sage.

Heat a large, heavy skillet over medium heat, and add 1 teaspoon olive oil. When oil is hot, add sausage mixture, and cook for 8 to 10 minutes, stirring and crumbling frequently.

Add apples and onions, stir well, reduce heat to medium-low, and cover. Cook for an additional 10 minutes or until sausage is cooked through and apples are fork tender. Taste for seasoning and add salt and/or freshly ground pepper as needed.

In a separate medium skillet, heat remaining olive oil over medium-high heat. Break eggs into pan and fry until yolk are done to taste.

To serve, place half of the hash onto each of 2 plates, and top each portion with 2 eggs.

Makes 2 servings.

Fresh Breakfast Scramble

This breakfast scramble is quick and easy, but loaded with flavor. Prepare the turkey bacon according to directions in the microwave, and you'll need only one pan to whip up this satisfying meal.

- 1 teaspoon olive oil
- ½ cup red bell pepper, diced
- ¼ cup sweet white onion, diced
- ¼ cup tomato, diced
- 2 tablespoons fresh parsley, chopped, plus additional sprigs to garnish
- ½ teaspoon salt
- ½ teaspoon freshly ground black pepper
- 4 large eggs, beaten
- 4 slices cooked turkey bacon, crumbled

Heat olive oil in a large, heavy skillet over medium heat. Add bell pepper and onion to skillet and stir occasionally, cooking for about 5 to 7 minutes or until onions are transparent.

Add tomato, parsley, salt, and pepper, and cook for another 2 minutes.

Increase heat to medium-high, and pour in the eggs. As soon as the eggs begin to set, sprinkle bacon crumbles over the eggs, distributing evenly.

Continue to cook, stirring constantly until eggs are fluffy and a little moist, about 2-5 minutes.

To serve, divide eggs between 2 plates, and garnish with a sprig of fresh parsley.

Makes 2 servings.

Southwestern Breakfast Skillet

This quick breakfast makes great use of leftover chicken and is an excellent dish to serve when you have company. Be sure to choose a salsa that has no added sugar.

- 1 tablespoon olive oil
- ½ cup sweet white onion, thinly sliced
- ¼ cup red bell pepper, diced
- ¼ cup yellow bell pepper, diced
- ½ cup white mushrooms, sliced
- 1 cup (about three breasts) cooked chicken, diced
- ¼ cup fresh parsley, chopped
- 8 large eggs, beaten
- 1 cup prepared salsa, warmed in microwave
- ½ cup sour cream
- Parsley or cilantro to garnish

In a large, heavy skillet, heat olive oil over medium-high heat. Add onion and red and yellow peppers, and sauté, stirring frequently, for 5 minutes or until onions are transparent.

Add mushrooms and cook for an additional 5 minutes.

Add chicken and parsley, distributing evenly through the mixture. Pour eggs over all, reduce heat to medium, and cover. Cook, covered, for about 6 to 7 minutes or until eggs are cooked through.

Slide eggs in 1 piece onto a cutting board, and use a knife or pizza wheel to slice into 4 wedges.

To serve, place each wedge on a plate, and top with ¼ cup salsa and a dollop of sour cream. Garnish with additional parsley or cilantro.

Makes 4 servings.

Apple-Cinnamon Protein Shake

This thick and creamy shake packs plenty of protein from the Greek yogurt and almond milk, plus healthy omega-3 fatty acid and fiber from the flax seed. Don't worry—you'll never taste the flax, but it will help you to stay full all morning.

- ½ cup vanilla-flavored Greek yogurt
- 1 cup unsweetened applesauce
- ½ cup vanilla-flavored almond milk
- 2 tablespoons sugar-free maple syrup
- 1 tablespoon ground flax seed
- 1 teaspoon cinnamon
- ¼ teaspoon nutmeg
- ½ cup ice cubes

In a blender, combine Greek yogurt, applesauce, almond milk, and sugar-free maple syrup. Blend until smooth and well combined.

Add flax seed, cinnamon, and nutmeg, and blend for about 30 seconds.

Add ice cubes and blend until smooth and thick.

To serve, pour into 2 (12-ounce) glasses. Garnish with an extra sprinkle of nutmeg, and drink immediately.

Makes 2 servings.

Special Steak and Eggs

Steak and eggs is an American institution, and this recipe offers a delicious new way to prepare it. The addition of red and orange bell peppers and fresh button mushrooms provides an antioxidant-loaded twist.

- 2 tablespoons olive oil, divided
- 1 red bell pepper, sliced ¼-inch thick
- 1 orange red pepper, sliced ¼-inch thick
- 1 medium onion, sliced ¼-inch thick
- 2 teaspoons salt, divided
- ½ pound whole, fresh button mushrooms
- 1 teaspoon freshly ground black pepper, divided
- 2 (4-5 ounce) sirloin steaks
- 4 large eggs

In a large, heavy skillet, heat 1 tablespoon olive oil over medium-high heat. Add red and orange bell peppers and onions, season with ½ teaspoon salt, and cook, stirring occasionally, for 5 minutes.

Add mushrooms and season with ½ teaspoon salt and ½ teaspoon freshly ground black pepper. Stirring often, cook for an additional 5 minutes, then remove vegetables to a covered platter to keep warm.

Increase heat to high and cook steaks in same pan, making sure to sear them well on both sides. Cook to desired doneness, season with remaining salt and pepper, and turn off heat. Cover pan to keep warm, and allow to rest for at least 5 minutes while cooking eggs.

In a separate heavy skillet, heat remaining olive oil, and fry eggs to desired doneness.

To serve, slice each steak and place on a plate. Top each portion with half of the vegetables, and serve the eggs alongside.

Makes 2 servings.

Lunch

Simply Good Chicken Noodle Soup

Few things are as comforting and filling as a steaming bowl of chicken noodle soup. You can simmer a good soup all day long, but this one has very nice flavor despite the short amount of cooking time. The shirataki noodles absorb flavors over time, so this soup is even better the next day.

- 1 tablespoon olive oil
- 2 fresh carrots, peeled and thinly sliced
- 1 small yellow onion, diced
- 1 rib of celery, thinly sliced
- ½ teaspoon salt
- ½ teaspoon freshly ground black pepper
- 1 teaspoon dried rosemary
- 1 teaspoon dried tarragon
- 6 cups low-sodium chicken broth
- 4 cooked chicken breasts, chopped
- 6 ounces frozen leaf spinach, thawed and well drained
- 2 (8-ounce) packages shirataki fettuccine noodles, rinsed and patted dry
- ¼ cup fresh parsley, chopped

In a large, heavy stockpot, heat olive oil over medium heat. Add carrots, onions, and celery, and cook, stirring occasionally, for 10 minutes.

Add salt, pepper, rosemary, and tarragon, stir well, and cook for 2 more minutes.

Pour in chicken broth, turn heat to medium-low, and cover. Let simmer for 10 minutes.

Add chicken and spinach and simmer, uncovered, for 5 minutes. Add noodles and stir well; cook until noodles are just heated through. Stir in parsley.

To serve, ladle into soup bowls.

Makes 6 servings.

Philly Lettuce Wraps

Sandwiches are something you have to rethink when on a wheat-free diet and are one of the first foods those starting out wonder how they'll replace. This gooey, melt-in-your-mouth sandwich is just as hearty and filling as the traditional version—you won't miss the bread.

- 1 teaspoon olive oil
- 1 clove garlic, crushed
- ½ cup green bell pepper, diced
- 1 medium white onion, thinly sliced
- ½ cup white mushrooms, sliced
- 12 slices (about 8 ounces) lean roast beef
- Salt and pepper to taste
- ½ cup shredded part-skim mozzarella cheese
- 4 large leaves romaine lettuce, washed and well dried

In a medium-sized heavy skillet, heat olive oil over medium heat. Add crushed garlic, bell pepper, and onion, and cook, stirring frequently, for about 5 minutes, or until peppers are just tender.

Add mushrooms and cook for 2 more minutes.

Slice roast beef into strips, and stir into the vegetable mixture. Using a large spoon or spatula, form the mixture into 2 small mounds. Season with salt and pepper to taste.

Sprinkle the shredded cheese onto the mounds. Cover the skillet and turn heat to low. Let sit for about 2 minutes or until cheese is melted.

While cheese melts, cut the ribs from 4 large leaves of romaine lettuce. Place 2 leaves "head to toe" to cover the spots from the missing ribs, overlapping about ⅓.

Place one mound of meat and veggies in the center of one pair of leaves. Fold the closest edge over the mound, working lengthwise. Fold the ends of the lettuce in toward the center, then finish rolling lengthwise.

To serve, cut each wrap in half diagonally.

Makes 2 servings.

Asian Noodle Bowl

Hitting an Asian restaurant for lunch isn't easy on a wheat-free diet, though it can be done. When you're in the mood for a hearty Asian dish, this noodle bowl can be prepared in mere minutes, and its vibrant flavors will satisfy your cravings.

- 1 teaspoon sesame oil
- 2 cloves garlic, crushed
- 1 teaspoon fresh ginger, grated
- 1 tablespoon low-sodium soy sauce
- 1 cup bok choy, chopped into 2-inch pieces
- 2 (8-ounce) packages shirataki ramen-style noodles, rinsed and dried

- ½ cup vegetable broth
- 1 tablespoon fresh cilantro, chopped
- 12 medium cooked shrimp, peeled and deveined
- 1 teaspoon hoisin sauce
- Sesame seeds to garnish

In a medium-heavy saucepan, heat sesame oil over medium heat. Add garlic, ginger, soy sauce, and bok choy, and cook, stirring frequently, for 3 minutes.

Add noodles and stir well to coat. Cook, continuing to stir frequently, for 2 more minutes.

Add broth, cilantro, and shrimp, and simmer for 3 to 4 minutes until shrimp is heated through. Stir in hoisin sauce.

To serve, use tongs to divide noodles, shrimp, and bok choy into deep bowls, and ladle the broth over each. Garnish with toasted sesame seeds if desired.

Makes 2 servings.

Mediterranean Grilled Chicken Salad

This salad is light and fresh, yet hearty enough to serve as a filling lunchtime meal. You can cook the chicken ahead of time over the weekend if you like. The chicken will keep well for up to three days in the refrigerator and be handy for making salads through the week.

- 1 teaspoon olive oil
- 8 raw, boneless, skinless chicken thighs
- 1 clove garlic, crushed
- 1 teaspoon dried rosemary
- 1 teaspoon dried thyme
- 1 teaspoon salt
- ½ teaspoon freshly ground black pepper
- 2 (6-ounce) cans of sliced black olives
- 3 cups fresh baby spinach leaves
- 1 medium red onion, thinly sliced
- 6 ounces goat cheese, cut into bite-sized pieces
- Prepared vinaigrette

In a large, heavy skillet, heat olive oil over medium-high heat.

Use a knife to cut down thicker portions of chicken thighs so they are of uniform thickness. Add garlic, rosemary, and thyme to skillet and stir.

Salt and pepper each thigh and place in skillet. Cook for about 5 minutes, then use tongs to turn over.

Cook for another 5 minutes, then add olives to pan, stirring to coat. Cook for 1 minute, then remove from heat.

Toss spinach, onion, and goat cheese in a large salad bowl. Add favorite vinaigrette dressing and toss again. Divide salad between 4 plates or bowls.

Cut chicken into bite-sized pieces, and add to each salad. Spoon olives over and serve.

Makes 4 servings.

Egg Salad in Avocadoes

When you're craving an egg salad sandwich from the deli, this stand-in is a delicious and healthy alternative. The larger, Florida variety of avocadoes are called for in this dish, rather than the smaller, softer Haas type.

- 1 medium, ripe avocado
- 1 teaspoon lemon juice
- 4 hard-boiled eggs, peeled and diced
- 1 stalk celery, thinly sliced
- ½ small white onion, diced
- ¼ cup sliced black olives
- ½ teaspoon salt
- ½ teaspoon freshly ground black pepper
- 1 teaspoon yellow mustard
- 2 tablespoons mayonnaise

Cut the avocado in half, peel, and remove the pit. Rub each half with the lemon juice to prevent browning, and set aside.

In a small mixing bowl, combine the eggs, celery, onions, olives, salt, and pepper until well blended.

In another small bowl, combine the mustard and mayonnaise, whisking well with a fork until smooth.

Mix the mayonnaise mixture into the egg mixture until well combined.

To serve, spoon the egg salad into the avocado halves.

Makes 2 servings.

Creamy Tomato Soup

This tomato soup takes only minutes to make, but the taste is far and above the flavor of any canned version. Slightly sweet, with a touch of garlic, it's a wonderful light soup for lunch.

- 1 teaspoon olive oil
- ¼ cup sweet white onion, diced
- 1 clove garlic, crushed
- 1 teaspoon salt
- ½ teaspoon freshly ground black pepper
- 2 (6-ounce) cans tomato paste
- 1 teaspoon Stevia In The Raw
- 1 (10-ounce) can diced tomatoes, unseasoned
- 2 cups milk
- 2 tablespoons Parmesan cheese
- Fresh parsley to garnish

In a medium-heavy saucepot, heat olive oil over medium-low heat. Add onion and garlic, and cook for 5 minutes, stirring frequently.

Add salt, pepper, and tomato paste, and stir until well combined. Stir in stevia.

Add diced tomatoes, stir to combine, then add in milk, blending well.

Cook for 5 minutes until heated through, taste for seasoning, and add salt and/or pepper as needed.

To serve, ladle into bowls, sprinkle with Parmesan cheese, and garnish with a sprig of fresh parsley.

Makes 4 servings.

Easy Spinach Quiche

If you've never made it, quiche only sounds intimidating. It's actually a very simple dish; uncomplicated enough to make in a hurry but sufficiently elegant and delicious for weekend company.

- 1 tablespoon extra-virgin olive oil
- 1 red bell pepper, chopped
- 1 medium red onion, chopped
- ½ teaspoon salt
- ½ teaspoon freshly ground black pepper
- 1 cup frozen chopped spinach, thawed and squeezed of excess water
- 8 large eggs
- 1 cup milk
- 1 cup shredded Swiss cheese

Preheat oven to 350 degrees.

Grease a 9-inch glass pie plate and set aside.

In a small, heavy skillet, heat olive oil over medium heat. Add peppers, onions, ½ teaspoon salt, and pepper to pan, and cook for 5 to 7 minutes, until peppers are slightly tender.

Add spinach to pan, and stir to coat. Cook for 3 minutes, stirring occasionally.

Meanwhile, in a medium mixing bowl, combine eggs and milk, and whisk well to combine.

Pour vegetable mixture into eggs, and add Swiss cheese. Pour all into the prepared pie plate and season with remaining salt.

Bake for 45 to 50 minutes or until completely set and slightly golden.

To serve, cut into wedges, and serve with a green salad.

Makes 8 servings.

Roasted Vegetable Soup

This soup is a wonderful way to savor the abundance of summer and its many flavors. It's easy to vary the particular taste by adding in whatever happens to be fresh from your garden or farmer's market. Note that this soup will keep well for an entire week.

- 2 medium zucchini, sliced in ¼-inch slices
- 2 summer squash, sliced in ¼-inch slices
- 1 red bell pepper, cut into 1-inch chunks
- 1 orange bell pepper, cut into 1-inch chunks
- 2 large white onions, peeled and cut into 1-inch chunks
- 2 tablespoons olive oil
- 1 teaspoon fresh rosemary
- 1 cup fresh green beans, trimmed and cut into 1-inch pieces
- 1 teaspoon fresh thyme
- ½ teaspoon turmeric
- 1 teaspoon salt
- ½ teaspoon freshly ground black pepper
- ¼ cup dry white wine
- 6 cups chicken or vegetable broth

Preheat oven to 400 degrees.

In a large bowl, toss zucchini, squash, red pepper, orange pepper, onion, and green beans in the olive oil to coat well.

Crumble rosemary and thyme together in a small bowl; add turmeric, salt, and pepper, and combine well. Pour over vegetables, and toss again to coat.

Spread vegetables evenly into a large, oven-safe skillet, and roast for 20 to 25 minutes until slightly fork tender. Remove vegetables from oven and scoop into a large, heavy stockpot.

Place skillet over medium-high heat. Once hot, add wine all at once and scrape bits from the surface of the pan. Add wine to the stockpot, and place the stockpot on the burner.

Bring pot to boil, add broth, and return to boil. Reduce heat to medium-low, cover, and simmer for 10 minutes.

To serve, ladle into deep bowls.

Makes 6 servings.

Shrimp and Avocado Platter

When you're in the mood for something light and fresh, this quick lunch is just the thing—it's also high in protein and heart-healthful fats.

- 1 tablespoon sea salt
- 1 teaspoon cider vinegar
- 1 pound (35-40) medium raw shrimp, peeled and deveined
- 1 large Florida avocado
- 2 large Granny Smith or other tart apple
- 1 tablespoon lemon juice
- 1 medium red onion, thinly sliced
- 1 teaspoon fresh cilantro, chopped
- 1 teaspoon fresh basil, chopped
- 1 pound packaged spring mix salad greens
- Prepared vinaigrette

Bring 6 cups of water to boil in a large pot. Add salt, vinegar, and shrimp, and cook just until shrimp are done, about 5 minutes. Pour into colander to drain.

Cut avocado in half, remove pit and skin, and slice into chunks. Place in a large salad bowl.

Peel and core apples, chop, and place in large bowl with avocadoes. Add lemon juice, and toss well to coat. Add onion, cilantro, and basil, and toss again.

Arrange salad greens on small plates, top with vegetable mixture, and arrange shrimp alongside. Dress with your favorite prepared vinaigrette.

Makes 4 servings.

Noodles with Ham and Peas

This is a hearty noodle dish that can be prepared in just a few minutes. The mixture of ham, peas, and cheese at the base of the sauce are a classic combination; the shirataki noodles make it wheat-free but just as delicious.

- 1 teaspoon olive oil
- 1 cup cooked ham, diced
- 1 medium cup white onion, diced
- ½ cup frozen peas, thawed
- 2 (8-ounce) packages of shirataki noodles, rinsed and dried
- 1 can cream of celery soup
- ¾ cup shredded Swiss cheese
- ½ cup unflavored almond milk
- 1 teaspoon freshly ground black pepper
- Salt to taste

In a large, heavy skillet, heat olive oil over medium heat. Add ham and onion, and cook just until onion is tender, about 5 minutes.

Add frozen peas and noodles, stirring well, and cook for 2 more minutes.

In a small bowl, mix soup, cheese, and milk, and pour into skillet. Add pepper and salt to taste.

Simmer for 2 minutes, stirring frequently, until cheese is melted.

Serve with a fresh green salad.

Makes 4 servings.

Dinner

Pecan-Crusted Flounder

Fish is a delicious and healthful alternative to red meat that can be prepared quickly and in an extensive variety of ways. This recipe delivers much of the flavor and texture of fried fish, but without the bread crumbs or batter.

- 1 large egg, beaten
- ½ cup unflavored almond milk
- 4 (6-8 ounce) fillets of fresh flounder
- 1½ cups pecan halves
- 1 teaspoon paprika
- 1 teaspoon garlic powder
- ½ cup fresh parsley, additional fresh parsley for garnish
- 1 teaspoon salt
- 1 teaspoon freshly ground black pepper
- 1 fresh lemon

Preheat oven broiler.

In a large, shallow dish, combine beaten egg and almond milk, mixing well. Lay fish fillets in milk mixture, turning once to coat. Let sit for 10 minutes.

Grease a baking sheet or shallow pan and set aside.

In a food processor, combine pecans, paprika, garlic powder, and parsley, and process until the mixture resembles a fine crumb similar to bread crumbs. Empty into a clean, shallow dish or onto a large plate.

Salt and pepper each fish fillet, then dredge each fillet on both sides, pressing down a bit into the crumbs to evenly coat the fillets.

Place each fish fillet onto the baking sheet, and place baking sheet on a rack about 6 inches from the broiler element.

Broil fish for 10 minutes, then gently turn each fillet with a spatula. Broil for another 5 to 7 minutes, until fish flakes easily with a fork.

Cut the lemon in half, and squeeze 1 half over all fillets. Slice the other half into 8 thin slices.

To serve, garnish each fillet with 2 overlapping slices of lemon and additional fresh parsley, if desired.

Makes 4 servings.

Pork Loin with Roasted Sweet Potato Strips

This is a great dish to serve for company or any time you want a comforting but elegant meal. When prepared this way, pork loin is especially lean, but full of flavor.

For the pork loin:
- 1 teaspoon paprika
- 1 teaspoon mild curry powder
- 1 teaspoon salt
- 1 teaspoon freshly ground black pepper
- 1 teaspoon ground sage
- 1 teaspoon dried rosemary
- 1 tablespoon olive oil
- 1 (1½-pound) pork loin

For the sweet potato strips:
- 1 teaspoon salt
- 1 teaspoon dried tarragon
- 1 teaspoon rosemary
- ½ teaspoon freshly ground black pepper
- 1 tablespoon olive oil
- 4 large sweet potatoes, peeled and cut into ½-inch thick strips

Preheat oven to 350 degrees.

In a 9 x 13-inch glass baking dish, combine paprika, curry powder, salt, pepper, sage, and rosemary, mixing well and spreading the mixture out as much as possible.

Heat the olive oil in a large, heavy skillet over medium-high heat.

Roll the pork loin in the spice mixture, turning to coat as evenly as possible. Rub any remaining spice mixture into the pork with your hands.

Sear the pork loin in the hot skillet for about 2 minutes per side, until evenly browned. Remove from heat and set aside.

Wipe any leftover spice mixture from the baking dish, and grease dish. Place the pork loin into the center of the dish and bake for 45 to 50 minutes or until a meat thermometer registers 140 degrees.

To prepare the sweet potato strips, combine the salt, tarragon, rosemary, and pepper in a small dish, mixing well.

Pour the olive oil into a large mixing bowl and toss the sweet potatoes, coating well. Add the spice mixture and toss again.

After the pork loin has been baking for 25 minutes, arrange the sweet potatoes around the pork loin, and return the dish to the oven. Bake until done.

Cover the pork loin with foil, and allow it to rest for 10 minutes before slicing.

To serve, spoon a portion of sweet potato strips onto the plate, and arrange sliced pork loin on top. This is wonderful served with a fresh, crisp salad.

Makes 4 servings.

Orange and Ginger Flank Steak Stir-Fry

Enjoy the flavors of a savory stir-fry dish using shirataki noodles in place of more traditional lo mein or rice noodles. These noodles absorb the delicious flavors of the sauce, so the dish tastes even better the following day.

- 1 pound flank steak, partially frozen
- 3 tablespoons low-sodium, wheat-free soy sauce
- 1 tablespoon orange juice concentrate, thawed
- ¼ cup sweet red wine
- 1 teaspoon sesame oil
- 1 teaspoon fresh ginger, crushed
- 1 clove fresh garlic, chopped
- ½ teaspoon freshly ground black pepper
- 1 cup fresh snow peas, strings removed
- 1 cup fresh bok choy, cut into 1-inch strips
- 1 cup red bell pepper, cut into strips
- 1 pound fresh, baby portobello mushrooms, sliced
- 1 tablespoon soy sauce mixed with 1 teaspoon fresh ginger, crushed
- 2 (8-ounce) packages ramen-style shirataki noodles, rinsed and dried
- 1 tablespoon fresh cilantro, chopped, for garnish

Slice the partially-frozen flank steak, against the grain, into ¼-inch thick slices. Place into a zippered plastic bag.

In a small bowl, combine soy sauce, orange juice concentrate, red wine, sesame oil, ginger, garlic, and pepper, and mix well. Pour into plastic bag, seal, and shake well to coat the steak pieces.

Place the plastic bag onto a plate, flattening the bag as much as possible, and refrigerate for 2 hours, turning occasionally.

Heat a large, heavy skillet over high heat and add steak. Cook for 3 to 4 minutes, stirring constantly.

Add snow peas, bok choy, bell pepper, and mushrooms, and pour red wine/ginger mixture over all. Add soy sauce/ginger mixture. Stir well to coat, then add noodles.

Cook, stirring frequently, for 2 to 3 minutes.

Ladle stir-fry into shallow bowls or onto plates, and garnish with fresh cilantro if desired.

Makes 4 servings.

Garlic and Herb Roasted Chicken

Few dishes are as iconic and beloved as a whole roasted chicken. This recipe makes a beautiful presentation that you'll be proud to serve guests—but don't wait for company to enjoy it.

- 1 whole roasting hen (4-5 pounds)
- 6 sprigs fresh rosemary
- 6 sprigs fresh thyme
- 6 sprigs fresh tarragon
- 4 cloves garlic, slightly crushed
- 1 tablespoon canola oil
- 1 teaspoon salt
- 1 teaspoon freshly ground black pepper
- ¼ cup fresh parsley, chopped to garnish

Preheat oven to 425 degrees.

Remove giblets and heart from inside the chicken, and set aside for making stock or some other use.

Gently loosen the skin from the breasts of the chicken, and place 3 sprigs each of the rosemary, thyme, and tarragon between the skin and the breast meat. Spread them out into a pretty arrangement, and then smooth the skin back down.

Tie the remaining herbs together with kitchen twine, and place together with garlic cloves into the cavity of the chicken.

Rub the canola oil all over the skin of the bird, then sprinkle salt and pepper both on the skin and in the cavity.

Place chicken on a poultry rack that has been set up inside a large roasting pan, and bake in the center of the oven for 20 minutes.

Reduce oven temperature to 375 degrees, and roast another 45 to 50 minutes, basting at least twice with the chicken's juices. Chicken is done when a meat thermometer inserted into the meatiest part of the thigh registers 165 degrees.

Remove the chicken from the oven, cover with foil, and allow it to sit for 10 minutes before carving.

To serve, carve breasts from the body, remove the legs, separate the drumstick from the thigh, and remove wings. Arrange the cuts on a serving platter, and sprinkle fresh parsley over all to garnish.

Makes 4 to 5 servings.

Shirataki Shrimp Scampi

There's no need to give up your favorite classic pasta dishes on the wheat-free diet. Shirataki noodles come in an angel hair-like variety that's perfect for many dishes, including this delicious take on shrimp scampi.

- 1 tablespoon olive oil
- 1 tablespoon salted butter
- 1½ pounds (35-40) raw medium shrimp, peeled and deveined
- 4 cloves fresh garlic, chopped
- ½ teaspoon sea salt
- ½ teaspoon freshly ground black pepper
- ¼ cup dry white wine
- ¼ cup clam juice
- 2 teaspoons fresh lemon juice
- 2 (8-ounce) packages of shirataki angel hair noodles, rinsed and dried
- ½ cup fresh chopped parsley
- 1 teaspoon fresh lemon zest

Combine olive oil and butter in a large, heavy skillet over medium-high heat. Once the oil and butter are quite hot, toss in the shrimp, and cook without turning for 2 minutes. Stir well, turning all of the shrimp, and add the garlic, salt, and pepper.

Cook shrimp for 2 to 3 minutes until pink, then add white wine, clam juice, and lemon juice. Stir well to coat the shrimp, and cook for 1 minute.

Use a slotted spoon to remove the shrimp to a plate. Add noodles and parsley to the pan, and stir again to combine. Cook for 1 more minute until noodles are heated through.

To serve, pour noodles and sauce onto a platter, and then top with shrimp. Garnish with lemon zest. Serve with freshly grated Parmesan cheese if desired.

Makes 4 servings.

Wine-Braised Cabbage Rolls

These cabbage rolls have an extra-hearty filling of ground beef, mushrooms, and mozzarella cheese that is especially satisfying. Gently oven-braised in a tomato-wine sauce, this dish is sure to please.

- 3 teaspoons salt, divided
- 8 large outer leaves of green cabbage, trimmed of ribs
- 1 teaspoon olive oil
- 2 cloves fresh garlic, crushed
- 1 green bell pepper, diced
- 1 large yellow onion, diced
- ½ pound fresh white mushrooms, chopped
- 1 teaspoon freshly ground black pepper
- 2 pounds lean ground beef
- 1½ cups shredded mozzarella cheese
- 1 teaspoon dried oregano
- 1 teaspoon dried marjoram
- 1 (6-ounce) can tomato paste
- ½ cup red wine
- 1 (10-ounce) can stewed tomatoes

In a large stockpot, bring 6 cups water to a boil. Add 1 teaspoon salt, and place cabbage leaves in pot. Boil for 5 minutes, remove from pot, and set aside.

Preheat oven to 325 degrees and grease a 9 x 13-inch casserole dish.

In a large, heavy skillet, heat olive oil over medium heat. Add garlic, peppers, onions, mushrooms, 1 teaspoon salt, and black pepper. Cook, stirring frequently, for 5 minutes. Remove from heat.

Place vegetables, ground beef, shredded cheese, oregano, and marjoram in a large mixing bowl and combine until well blended.

Working with one cabbage leaf at a time, spoon ⅛ of the meat mixture onto a cabbage leaf, placing it about 3 inches in from the closest edge. Fold the closest edge over the meat, fold each in toward the center, and continue rolling. Place seam side down in prepared casserole. Continue until all 8 packets have been rolled.

In a medium bowl, combine tomato paste, remaining salt, and red wine. Mix well until smooth, then add stewed tomatoes, and blend well.

Pour tomato mixture over the cabbage rolls, and bake for 45 to 50 minutes, or until a meat thermometer inserted into the center of a roll registers 165 degrees.

To serve, place 2 cabbage rolls on each plate, and spoon additional sauce over each.

Makes 4 servings.

Hearty Beef and Vegetable Soup

This soup will satisfy the healthiest appetite, especially on cooler days. It keeps very well in the refrigerator or freezer, so make a double batch to have some on hand for convenient lunches as well.

- 1 pound lean ground beef
- 1 teaspoon salt
- 1 teaspoon freshly ground black pepper
- 4 large carrots, peeled and diced
- 1 stalk celery, thinly sliced
- 1 large yellow onion, diced
- 2 tablespoons tomato paste
- ½ pound button mushrooms, sliced
- 4 cups beef stock or beef broth
- 1 tablespoon Worcestershire sauce
- 1 bay leaf
- 1 teaspoon dried parsley, plus additional fresh parsley to garnish

In a large, heavy stockpot, cook ground beef over medium heat, crumbling frequently with a spatula, for about 5 minutes.

Add salt, pepper, carrots, celery, and onion, and cook for another 5 minutes, stirring occasionally.

Stir in tomato paste until well blended, and then add mushrooms, beef stock, Worcestershire, bay leaf, and parsley. Bring to a simmer, then reduce heat to low, and cover.

Simmer for 30 minutes or until carrots are done. Remove bay leaf before serving.

To serve, ladle into soup bowls. If desired, garnish with fresh parsley.

Makes 4 servings.

Shrimp and Asparagus Pasta

This recipe is extremely quick to pull together when using precooked shrimp. It's a great dish for busy weeknights and tastes light and fresh—a perfect summer meal. If you prefer to use fresh shrimp, it'll take only another ten minutes or so to prepare.

- 1 tablespoon salted butter
- 1 teaspoon extra-virgin olive oil
- 1 clove garlic, crushed
- 1 pound fresh asparagus, ends trimmed and cut into 1-inch pieces
- ½ red bell pepper, diced
- 1 teaspoon salt
- ½ teaspoon white pepper
- 1 pound (34–40) cooked shrimp, peeled and deveined
- 2 (8-ounce) packages of penne-style shirataki noodles, rinsed
- ½ fresh lemon
- 1 tablespoon toasted sesame seeds to garnish

In a large, heavy skillet, heat the butter and oil. When the butter has melted, add the garlic, asparagus, bell pepper, salt, and white pepper. Reduce heat to medium-low and cover.

Cook vegetables, stirring often, for 10 minutes, or until peppers and asparagus are just tender.

Add shrimp and noodles, stirring well, and cook just until heated through.

To serve, spoon onto plates, and top each serving with a squeeze of fresh lemon juice. Garnish with sesame seeds.

Makes 4 servings.

Spicy Beef and Peppers

This recipe will appeal to those who like a bit of heat in their meal, but it's not too spicy for more sensitive palates. If you have leftovers, reheat and wrap in lettuce leaves for a low-carb lunch.

- 1 pound sirloin steak, partially frozen
- 1 tablespoon plus 1 teaspoon olive oil
- 1 tablespoon wheat-free soy sauce
- 1 teaspoon fresh ginger, chopped
- 2 cloves fresh garlic, crushed
- ½ teaspoon black pepper
- ½ teaspoon red pepper flakes
- 1 red bell pepper, cut into strips
- 1 yellow bell pepper, cut into strips
- 1 green pepper, cut into strips
- 1 medium onion, thinly sliced
- 1 pound whole button mushrooms

Slice the sirloin steak against the grain while still partially frozen. Place into a zippered plastic bag, and add 1 teaspoon olive oil, soy sauce, ginger, garlic, black pepper, and red pepper flakes.

Seal, shake well to coat the steak strips, and place on a plate. Refrigerate for 1 hour, turning periodically.

Heat 1 tablespoon olive oil in a large heavy skillet or wok over high heat. Add beef, including marinade, to the pan, and cook for 2 minutes, stirring constantly.

Add bell peppers, onions, and mushrooms, and cook for another 3 to 4 minutes until peppers are just a bit tender.

To serve, spoon over shirataki noodles or brown rice.

Makes 4 servings.

Dilly-Orange Sole Steamed in Foil

This quick fish dish takes just fifteen minutes to cook, and the cleanup couldn't be easier. You can do this on the grill if you like, too. Sole is used in this recipe, but feel free to substitute any light fish, such as tilapia. Choose fillets that are about one-inch thick to avoid overcooking them.

- 4 (6-8 ounce) fillets fresh or thawed sole, about 1-inch thick
- 2 Valencia oranges, unpeeled, thinly sliced
- 8 sprigs fresh dill
- 4 sprigs fresh basil
- 1 teaspoon salt
- ½ teaspoon freshly ground black pepper
- 2 tablespoons butter, cut into 4 pieces
- Salt and freshly ground pepper, to taste

Preheat oven to 375 degrees.

Cut 4 sheets of aluminum foil about 12 inches long, and lay them out on a work surface. Grease upper side of each.

Place 1 fish fillet on the left side of 1 sheet of foil, about 1 inch from the left edge. Place 3 or 4 slices of orange along the top of the fillet, and top with 2 sprigs of dill and 1 of basil. Sprinkle with salt and pepper, and add 1 piece of butter.

Fold the right half of the foil over the fish, and roll the edges of the foil inward, creating an edge similar to pie crust. Place on a baking sheet.

Repeat for the remaining 3 fillets, and bake for 15 minutes.

To serve, place 1 packet on each plate, crimped side up. Allow guests to slit open packets at the table.

Makes 4 servings.

Dessert

No-Flour Rich Chocolate Cake

Flourless chocolate cakes have long been a favorite dessert in fine restaurants, and they're much easier to make than their taste would suggest. This recipe is deceptively simple and a real treat for chocolate lovers. For sweetening in this dish, stevia extract is used, as the liquid performs better in baked goods than does the granulated version.

- ½ cup plus 1 tablespoon unsweetened cocoa powder, divided
- ½ cup salted butter
- 4 (1-ounce squares) unsweetened baking chocolate
- 1 cup Stevia Extract In The Raw
- 3 large eggs, beaten
- 1 teaspoon vanilla extract
- 1 teaspoon cinnamon

Preheat oven to 300 degrees.

Grease the bottom of an 8-inch round baking pan and lightly dust with 1 tablespoon of cocoa powder. Tap pan over sink to remove any excess cocoa powder.

In a small saucepan, bring 2 cups water to simmer over medium heat. Place butter and unsweetened chocolate in a large metal bowl and place over simmering water. Melt slowly, stirring frequently, then remove from heat.

Stir in stevia, remaining cocoa powder, eggs, vanilla extract, and cinnamon, and stir just until blended. Pour into cake pan.

Pour warm water from saucepan into a 9 x 13-inch or larger baking pan or casserole dish, just until water reaches halfway up the sides of the pan. Place on middle rack of preheated oven, and place cake pan into the larger pan.

Bake for 30 minutes, and carefully remove cake pan from the water bath. Allow to cool in the pan for 15 minutes, then carefully turn out onto a wire rack to finish cooling. Slice into 8 pieces once completely cooled.

Serve slightly warmed or at room temperature with a light dusting of cocoa powder on top.

Store leftover cake in the refrigerator in a tightly covered container.

Makes 8 servings.

Pecan-Apple Tart

Ground nuts make a delicious stand-in for flour-based pie crusts. While they don't hold their shape quite as well as traditional crusts, nut crusts add an extra layer of flavor that can't be beat. This is a delicious dessert to serve in the fall, when apples are at their peak of flavor.

For the crust:
- 1½ cups pecan halves
- ½ cup Stevia In The Raw
- 1 teaspoon ground cinnamon
- 1 teaspoon ground nutmeg
- ¾ cup salted butter, melted
- 1 large egg, beaten
- 1 teaspoon vanilla extract

For the filling:
- 4 Granny Smith or Gala apples, peeled and cut in ¼-inch slices
- 1 teaspoon ground cinnamon
- 2 tablespoons Stevia In The Raw
- ½ teaspoon salt
- 2 tablespoons salted butter, melted

Preheat oven to 325 degrees.

Place pecans, stevia, cinnamon, and nutmeg in a food processor, and process until finely chopped. Add melted butter, egg, and vanilla, and pulse until mixture resembles a fine crumble.

Press mixture into a 9-inch pie plate, forming a crust that reaches halfway up the sides of the pie plate. Set aside.

In a large bowl, toss apple slices in cinnamon, stevia, and salt until fairly well coated. Pour melted butter over the apples and toss again.

Pour apple filling into pie plate, and bake for 30 minutes or until apples are fork tender and golden.

Cool completely before cutting into 8 slices. Crust will be crumbly.

Store leftover tart in the refrigerator for up to 3 days in a tightly covered container.

Makes 8 servings.

Creamy Coconut Rice Pudding

Few desserts are as satisfying as a creamy dish of rice pudding. This recipe uses both coconut and almond milk to give it a slightly exotic flavor without sacrificing any of the richness.

- 1½ cups coconut milk
- ¾ cup short-grain rice
- 1½ cups unflavored almond milk, divided
- ⅓ cup Stevia In The Raw
- ½ teaspoon salt
- 1 teaspoon ground cinnamon
- ½ teaspoon ground nutmeg
- 1 large egg, beaten
- ½ cup raisins
- 1 tablespoon butter
- ½ teaspoon vanilla extract
- ¼ cup toasted coconut flakes

In a medium saucepan, bring coconut milk to a boil over medium heat. Stir in rice, reduce heat to low, and cover. Simmer for 20 minutes.

Add 1 cup of the almond milk, stevia, salt, cinnamon, and nutmeg. Simmer over medium heat, stirring occasionally, for 20 minutes. Pudding will thicken as at cooks.

Add the remaining almond milk, egg, raisins, butter, and vanilla, stirring well. Simmer for 5 minutes, stirring frequently.

To serve, spoon into 4 bowls, and top each serving with ¼ of the toasted coconut. This dessert is best served warm.

Makes 4 servings.

Warm Peach Parfaits

This dessert is fresh and light yet packs a nice dose of protein from the Greek yogurt. It's a delicious way to end a meal, especially in summer. Choose peaches that are slightly underripe, as ripe peaches can become too mushy.

- 4 white or yellow peaches, peeled and sliced
- 2 tablespoons lemon juice
- 1 teaspoon nutmeg
- 1 cup vanilla-flavored Greek yogurt
- 4 tablespoons chopped black walnuts
- 4 teaspoons Stevia In The Raw
- 2 tablespoons butter, cut into 4 slices

Preheat oven broiler.

In a medium mixing bowl, combine peaches, lemon juice, and nutmeg, and toss with hands to coat well. Divide peaches among 4 (½-cup) greased ramekins.

Top each ramekin with ¼ cup Greek yogurt, then 1 tablespoon black walnuts.

Sprinkle each ramekin with 1 teaspoon stevia, and place 1 slice of butter in the center of each.

Place ramekins onto a cookie sheet, and broil for 3 to 4 minutes or just until topping is slightly golden.

Allow to cool for 10 minutes before serving.

Makes 4 servings.

Individual Pumpkin-Pecan Custards

This recipe is extremely quick and easy and will satisfy your cravings for pumpkin pie at any time of year. You can make these ahead of time if you like; they'll keep for up to three days in the refrigerator if covered with plastic wrap. Allow them to come to room temperature before serving.

- 1 (15-ounce) can of plain pumpkin
- 2 large eggs, beaten
- 1 cup unflavored almond milk
- 2 tablespoons liquid stevia extract
- 2 teaspoons ground cinnamon
- 1 teaspoon ground ginger
- ½ teaspoon ground nutmeg
- 4 tablespoons chopped pecans

Preheat oven to 375 degrees.

Grease 6 (1-cup) ramekins, and place on a cookie sheet.

In a large mixing bowl, combine pumpkin, eggs, almond milk, and stevia extract. Stir well with a wooden spoon, or mix on low speed with a hand mixer until blended.

Add cinnamon, ginger, and nutmeg, and stir well or blend for 1 minute on low speed.

Divide evenly between ramekins, and top with chopped pecans.

Bake at 375 degrees for 15 minutes, then reduce heat to 300 degrees, and bake for 20 more minutes or until set.

Cool to room temperature, and serve in the ramekins.

Makes 6 servings.

Creamy Espresso Mousse

Chocolate mousse is a favorite, classic dessert, but it's usually made with heavy cream and a good deal of sugar. This recipe contains far less fat and substitutes stevia for sugar, but it's so rich and creamy that no one will realize.

- ½ cup coconut milk
- 2 large eggs, beaten
- 8 (1-ounce) squares unsweetened baking chocolate, roughly chopped
- ½ cup brewed espresso
- 6 tablespoons liquid stevia extract
- 4 tablespoons coconut oil
- 1 teaspoon vanilla extract
- 4 small sprigs fresh mint to garnish

Place coconut milk in a medium saucepan and heat over medium-high heat just until simmering. Remove from heat.

Pour just a few tablespoons of the hot coconut milk into the beaten eggs to temper them, stirring rapidly, then pour egg mixture back into the saucepan. Mix well, and cook for 1 minute, stirring constantly. Remove from heat.

Put chopped chocolate into a medium mixing bowl, and pour hot coconut milk mixture over the chocolate. Stir until chocolate is just melted.

Add espresso, stevia extract, coconut oil, and vanilla, and then pour all into a blender.

Blend at high speed for about 1 minute until well mixed and smooth.

Divide mixture between 4 dessert glasses or ramekins, cover with plastic wrap, and chill for 4 to 6 hours to set.

Serve cold, garnishing each serving with a sprig of mint.

Makes 4 servings.

Strawberry-Pineapple Sorbet

This sorbet is simple and quick to make and rivals that of your favorite ice cream store. If you'd like to vary the flavors, try substituting lemon juice for the lime or unsweetened white grape juice for the pineapple.

- ⅔ cup unsweetened pineapple juice
- 2 pounds fresh strawberries, washed and hulled
- 2 tablespoons fresh lime juice
- 2 teaspoons liquid stevia extract
- 1 teaspoon lime zest
- Mint leaves or fresh sliced strawberries to garnish, if desired

Combine all ingredients in a blender, and blend on high until smooth.

Pour into a round or metal cake pan (do not use a nonstick pan), cover with plastic wrap, and place in the freezer for 4 hours.

Scoop sorbet mixture back into blender, blend again for about 1 minute, and pour back into pan.

Refreeze for 2 hours, and then use an ice cream scoop to spoon into individual dessert dishes. Garnish with mint leaves or fresh, sliced strawberries if desired.

Makes 6 servings.

Peanut Butter-Raisin Cookies

If you thought you'd have to live without cookies on a wheat-free diet, this delicious recipe should make you very happy. Flourless cookies don't freeze very well, so it's best to eat these while they're fresh.

- 1 cup chunky peanut butter
- 2 tablespoons liquid stevia extract
- 1 large egg, beaten
- 1 teaspoon milk
- 1 teaspoon baking soda
- ½ cup raisins

Preheat oven to 325 degrees, and line a cookie sheet with parchment paper.

In a large mixing bowl, combine peanut butter, stevia, egg, and milk. Using a hand mixer, beat on low speed for 2 minutes until smooth.

Add baking soda, and beat for 1 minute on low speed. Stir in raisins, and mix by hand until well incorporated.

Grease hands, then spoon out cookie dough in rounded teaspoons, and roll in both hands to form a ball. Grease hands again as needed to keep dough from sticking.

Place each ball on the cookie sheet, and flatten gently with a fork.

Bake for 6 to 8 minutes, remove from the oven, and slide off cookie sheet to cool.

These cookies store well in an airtight container for up to 3 days.

Makes 2 dozen cookies.

Very Berry Dessert

If you're looking for a light dessert, look no farther than this fresh-tasting, easy-to-make combination of strawberries and raspberries. The berry mixture tastes even better the second day, so feel free to make in advance, and assemble when you're ready to serve.

- 1 cup fresh strawberries, hulled and sliced
- 1 cup fresh red raspberries
- 1 teaspoon Stevia In The Raw
- 1 teaspoon fresh lime juice
- 1 cup vanilla-flavored Greek yogurt
- 1 teaspoon lime zest
- 4 fresh mint leaves to garnish

In a large, zippered freezer bag, combine the strawberries, raspberries, and stevia. Shake well to coat the berries, then place the bag onto a platter, and flatten before placing into the refrigerator.

Chill the berries for 2 hours, shaking once after the first hour to mix the berries.

Pour the berries into a medium mixing bowl. Add the lime juice, and stir well to blend.

Divide the berries into 4 individual dessert dishes, and top each with ¼ cup Greek yogurt.

Sprinkle each cup with ¼ of the lime zest, garnish with mint, and serve.

Makes 4 servings.

Frothy Chocolate Milkshakes

Few desserts are as beloved as a thick and creamy chocolate milkshake. Unlike the type you'll get at an ice cream store or fast food restaurant, this shake is actually good for you. The almond milk gives it a hint of nuttiness that's extra delicious.

- 4 tablespoons cocoa powder
- 2 tablespoons hot water
- 2 cups vanilla-flavored almond milk
- ½ teaspoon liquid stevia extract
- 6-8 ice cubes

In a small plastic container, combine cocoa powder, hot water, and stevia. Cover tightly and shake vigorously until the cocoa is well blended.

In a blender, combine almond milk and cocoa mixture, and blend on high speed for 30 seconds.

Add ice cubes and blend again until thick and creamy.

To serve, pour into 2 tall glasses, and drink immediately.

Makes 2 servings.

CONCLUSION

Making the decision to go on a wheat-free diet is one of the best health decisions you will ever make. Not only will you see wonderful improvements to your current health, but you also reduce the risks to your future health. Losing weight and eating foods that nourish your body and provide all the essential nutrients will give you renewed energy and a renewed interest in activities that may have been difficult or uncomfortable before.

Knowing you've done something truly important for your health, even when the process was difficult, can give you a new confidence and a desire to try other exciting challenges. You'll also be setting a healthful example for your friends and family as you learn new ways of eating. Enjoy the transition to your lifestyle. Enjoy the benefits even more!

REFERENCES

Centers for Disease Control and Prevention. 2012. *Diabetes Report Card 2012*. Atlanta, GA: Centers for Disease Control and Prevention, US Department of Health and Human Services.

Cheng, Jianfeng, Pardeep S. Brar, Anne R. Lee, and Peter H. R. Green. 2010. "Body Mass Index in Celiac Disease: Beneficial Effect of a Gluten-Free Diet." *Journal of Clinical Gastroenterology* 44 (April): 267–71.

Cordain, Loren. 2002. "Archeological Dermatology.": 1584–90.

Costa, Erminio, and Marci Trabucchi. 1980. *Advances in Biochemical Psychopharmacology*. New York: Raven Press.

Davis, William. 2011. *Wheat Belly: Lose the Wheat, Lose the Weight, and Find Your Path Back to Health*. Pennsylvania: Rodale Books.

Frassetto. L., R. C. Morris, Jr., D. E. Sellmeyer, K. Todd, and A. Sebastian. 2001. "Diet, Evolution and Aging." *European Journal of Nutrition* 40 (October): 200–213.

Hadjivassiliou, Marios, Richard Grünewald, Basil Sharrack, David Sanders, Alan Lobo, Clare Williamson, Nicola Woodroofe, Nicholas Wood, and Aelwyn Davies-Jones. 2003. "Gluten Ataxia in Perspective: Epidemiology, Genetic Susceptibility and Clinical Characteristics." *Brain* 126 (3): 685–91.

Harvard School of Public Health. February 2007. "Abdominal Fat and What to Do About It." *Harvard Medical School Family Health Guide*, accessed November 14, 2012, http://www.health.harvard.edu/fhg/updates/Abdominal-fat-and-what-to-do-about-it.shtml.

Ludvigsson, Jonas F., Scott M. Montgomery, Anders Ekbom, Lena Brandt, and Fredrik Granath. 2009. "Small-Intestine Histopathology and Mortality Risk in Celiac Disease." *The Journal of the American Medical Association* 302 (September): 1171–78.

Miyagi, S., N. Iwama, T. Kawabata, and K. Hasegawa. 2003. "Longevity and Diet in Okinawa, Japan: The Past, Present and Future." *Asia-Pacific Journal of Public Health* 15: 3–9.

Murray, Joseph A., Tureka Watson, Beverlee Clearman, and Frank Mitros. 2004. "Effect of a Gluten-Free Diet on Gastrointestinal Symptoms in Celiac Disease." *The American Journal of Clinical Nutrition* 79 (April): 669–73.

NDIC (National Diabetes Information Clearinghouse). October 2008. *Insulin Resistance and Prediabetes*, accessed November 15, 2012. http://diabetes.niddk.nih.gov/dm/pubs/insulinresistance/#symptoms.

Shewry, P. R. 2009. "Wheat." *Journal of Experimental Botany* 60 (6): 1537–53.

Song, Xiao, Zhongfy Ni, Yingyin Yao, Yinhong Zhang, and Qixin Sun. January 2009. "Identification of Differentially Expressed Proteins between Hybrid and Parents in Wheat (*Triticum aestivum L.*) Seedling Leaves." *Theoretical Applied Genetics* 118 (January): 213–25.

Whiteley, Paul, Demetrious Haricopos, Ann-Mari Knivsberg, Karl Ludvig Reichelt, Sarah Parlar, Judith Jacobsen, Anders Seim, Lennart Pedersen, Maja Schondel, and Paul Shattock. 2010. "The ScanBrit Randomised, Controlled, Single-Blind Study of a Gluten- and Casein-Free Dietary Intervention for Children with Autism Spectrum Disorders." *Nutritional Neuroscience* 13 (April): 87–100.

Wilson, Dr. Ayla. December 5, 2011. "The Wheat Belly: Diabetes and Accelerated Aging." *Fitness Goop*, accessed November 14, 2012. http://www.fitnessgoop.com/2011/12/the-wheat-belly-diabetes-and-accelerated-aging.

Zioudrou, C., R. A. Streaty, and W. A. Klee. 1979. "Opioid Peptides Derived from Food Proteins. The Exorphins." *The Journal of Biological Chemistry* 254 (April): 2446–49.

Made in the USA
San Bernardino, CA
24 January 2014